The B12 Deficiency Survival Handbook

Copyright © 2014 by Regev Elya.

Disclaimer

I0439311

Table of Contents

Publisher's Preface
by Regev Elya

Let me get straight to the point, fellas. I'm super-proud to be introducing this book. B12 started as a particular interest of mine back in the days when I practised veganism (I now don't) and it ended up being quite a passion.

What started as a few highly-researched articles on my site ended up being this book. I received a good amount of emails, comments and responses which I found very exhausting to be answering each and every time. Then the idea struck.

"Why won't I just create the perfect resource for this vitamin?"

That's how this book was born.

I knew my limitations though. I knew what B12 does but I needed some reinforcement when it comes to the biochemical process behind it. I then collaborated with Dr. *Aqsa Ghazanfar*, who brought a lot of credibility and top-notch research abilities to the table. With plenty of specialist help and on the shoulders of giant scientists, we managed to create this resource.

The book you are about to read is the direct result of hours and hours and of sometimes-enlightening-sometimes-frustrating research, separating the junk from the real legit science. We owe our thanks to some great Ph.Ds who helped with it, and we're very confident it's going to solve all your B12 issues.

Time to de-construct the mystery behind this vitamin to small, manageable, easy-to-understand pieces.

With no further ado, let's give the reins to Dr. Ghazanfar. She's the one who did the heavy lifting, I'm just the architect and editor.

Chapter 1: Introduction

Why a B12 Deficiency Book
If someone asked me 15 years ago to write about something that in my opinion deserves immediate medical attention, I would have probably chosen to write about heart disease or cancer.

My choice wouldn't be based on the fact that these diseases are the leading causes of death, or that they are relatively incurable once they reach a particular stage. If I were to write based on those, I would probably collect some morose data and make a book out of it.

If good enough, it would end up with research institutions or land me a good job. Those are not the accomplishments I wish to make when I write about something. I want to write material that really makes a difference.

Whenever I find out about something that could change people's lives or prevent them from acquiring a disease, I simply write about it. Making the right diagnosis is just a small part of our job as doctors. But it's not enough for me, especially when I find out alarming facts about something as simple as a vitamin.

The vitamin I'm talking about is B12. So what 'alarming' statistics did I come across? According to the *Agricultural Research Service of the United Sates*, it is estimated that 40 percent of people between 26 and 83 years of age have B12 levels in the plasma which are in the lower normal range. [1]

This range is what's followed in the labs but many individuals experience symptoms at these values. What's even worse is that low B12 levels are almost equally common amongst the youth and the elderly.Vitamin B12 deficiency is found in approximately 40 percent of those above the age of 60 years.

'So what?' you're saying, 'There are numerous other diseases that require attention!'; this seems to be a trivial issue, doesn't it? Absolutely not! Don't mistake these vital statistics to be mere data – here's why vitamin B12 deficiency can rightly be called an epidemic[2] which requires immediate attention:

- If 40% of the elderly population suffers from a B12 deficiency and symptoms of numerous diseases attributed to ageing (such as Alzheimer's, decreased cognitive function, dementia and lethargy) mimic the symptoms of B12 deficiency, then many people above the age of 60 might as well have a very easily curable vitamin deficiency!

- How could it be that simple? Wouldn't doctors know if it's a B12 deficiency? No. That's because this topic is not covered well in medical schools which is why many doctors do not test for it routinely. I know this because I'm a doctor myself.

- What's even worse is that the lab values of normal levels of B12 in the plasma are too low. Many people experience symptoms even when their B12 levels are within normal limits. The former fact is the main reason why such a large amount of people suffering from this easily curable disease are never being diagnosed with it. Damnation.

These 'deficiencies' in the health care system have been recognised by numerous doctors and those specialising in the treatment of B12 deficiency. However, awareness of this issue still does not exist on a fairly large scale and a lot has to be done if we are to successfully rid ourselves of this problem.

The first step is always from the patient whenever it comes to the diagnosis and treatment of a disease. If a patient does not recognise his own symptoms and report to a doctor, there isn't much that can be done about his disease.

Therefore, do not ignore the symptoms that this disease causes, however mild they might be, and consult your doctor about the required tests as well as the treatment options.

If you're not satisfied with the explanation you get, do not delay a consultation with a specialist who treats B12 deficiency specifically since the treatment is ridiculously simple and untreated disease could turn your life upside down.

Don't believe me? The chapters that follow will definitely clarify any doubts you have. So until then, let's read on.

Who Am I?

If you're concerned about that, well and good. If not, I'm worried about you. When it comes to your health, do not believe just about anything you hear or read – check the qualifications of the author and always look up the references they have given in context to whatever they have written. Nothing in science is acceptable without proof.

So who am I? I'm a medical doctor, not a nutritionist or a nutrition scientist. But why am I writing this book and not some 'specialist'?

That's because scientists have already written a couple of books and done a lot of research already – that hard work has just not reached people like us (yet).

When I read statistics regarding vitamin B12, I started looking up why it remains undiagnosed and how it could affect literally every organ of the body. You see, we doctors aren't exactly taught all the aspects of nutritional deficiencies and interestingly, this particular deficiency can make us flip through the textbooks of just about any speciality!

I read paper after paper of research carried out on B12 – only to discover that most of us don't have a darn clue how this deficiency is affecting millions of people and could be the possible cause of incurable conditions such as Alzheimer and contributes to heart disease amongst the other problems it leads to.

That was enough to make me and Regev decide we had to let people know – SOMETHING had to be done. With that notion began the creation of this book. There is no use of the massive research that specialists and dedicated doctors have carried out if it's not shared with you – whether you are a concerned mother, an individual in his 50's worried about his health or just a keen fitness freak.

That's the motive behind the creation of this book. It should not be taken as the sole source for diagnosis so consult your doctor if what you read here makes you think you might be suffering from a vitamin B12 deficiency. After all, that's what we're trying to accomplish through this book. Even if it gets one B12 deficient person to his or her doctor in time to be saved from permanent damage to his body, I would consider our mission accomplished.

Therefore, go to your doctor in time and ask them to get your tests done. If you're not satisfied, consult a specialist. This condition might be ridiculously easy to treat but it might not be that easy to diagnose.

Structure and Function of B12

The term 'Vitamin B12' is actually a single name given to a group of compounds known as the '*Cobalamins*'. All of them contain Cobalt and possess the 'Corrin' ring in their chemical structure due to which they are also referred to as the '*Corrinoids.*'

Not all of these compounds have the same activity as the B12 we talk about when referring to how the human body utilises this vitamin. Interestingly, this group of chemically related compounds even contains some substances which act as antagonists to the type of cobalamins the human body uses.

The metabolism of this vitamin in our body is complex, involving multiple stages and pathways. Once it has been taken up by the body, it begins its function by working alongside three major enzymes of the body, the end result being the production of DNA, red cell synthesis, conversion of carbohydrates into energy, and more.

Each of these functions will be described separately in the book, but to sum up - you should know that this vitamin passes multiple steps to finally get into your blood and has a complex metabolism which is why a minor problem at any of those metabolic steps can cause a deficiency.

It is involved in almost all the cells of your body and affects things as minor as your mood to organs as major as your brain. It might sound like big words, but it's all going to be clear soon. Just know that B12 is no joke, it's a serious matter.

Where Does Vitamin B12 Actually Come From?

Vitamins are unique because they are not synthesised in adequate amounts in our bodies and we need a particular amount of each vitamin in order to maintain our health. They cannot be stored in sufficient amounts which means you have to make sure you you get the required daily amounts of each vitamin or else, the signs and symptoms of its deficiency will start showing up, putting your health at risk. Not so sexy.

Vitamin B12 is considered to be the most unique in this group of nutrients. That is because the human body has the ability to store amounts of B12 that can last for several years.

Interestingly but rather unfortunately, absolutely no animals or plants are capable of producing this vitamin on their own. It is solely made by bacteria and its best sources are of animal origin – plants do not need it and thus don't store it.

The animal sources are thus the stored form of the vitamin, giving us a rich supply of B12. That definitely sounds like bad news for the vegans[3]. In case you're not a vegan and what you just read made a self-satisfied grin appear on your face, don't think only vegans can be affected.

Like I said earlier, B12 has a complex, step-by-step metabolism. A problem at any of these steps could cause a deficiency. Therefore, even if John Smith consumes the right amount of this vitamin, he could still develop its deficiency owing to problems within his body that do not let the vitamin get absorbed.

Of course, there's a long list of common as well uncommon conditions that can lead to such an issue but all those problems will be dealt with one by one, slowly unravelling the physiology and subsequent pathology of this truly beneficial nutrient.

Why is B12 Such a Problem In The Western World

I'm guessing you think you already know the answer to this one, provided you live in a modern place with plenty of vegan activity around. You're partially correct. Don't think I'm being unfair, here's the remaining half I didn't mention earlier:

People residing in the west, in addition to having a greater tendency to adopt vegetarian diets, are also prone to developing those conditions that can cause malabsorption in the gastrointestinal tract - resulting in reduced or no uptake of B12, eventually resulting in a deficiency. And this is a much bigger problem than proper vegetarianism.

There are multiple theories as to why particular populations are prone to developing particular diseases. For example, studies and research has related the traditional diets in Japan with the high incidence of stomach cancer in this country.[4]

Similarly, it is proposed that since people in the western world have better living conditions than those in the developing world, their immune systems are not developed well enough (due to their hygienic practices and consequent non-exposure to germs, dust, etc).

Due to this failure to develop properly, their immune systems start attacking their own bodies, thus the higher incidence of immune-mediated diseases such as asthma, Crohn's disease, Ulcerative Colitis, Autoimmune gastritis, etc. In simple terms, the body launches an immune response to stimuli which shouldn't normally make it do so (such as dust and pollen, for example).

There is a multitude of such theories but none have been proven so far. The discussion of why these diseases occur will not be a part of this book (although I would waste no time in writing about any of these if I ever come across an answer).

What's more important is how they can affect B12 metabolism since this is the issue that can be solved quickly and inexpensively, costing no more than a few dollars a month in some cases.

Imagine just how life could change if the decrease in cognition due to so-called 'ageing' could be prevented by attaining the rightly needed amount of B12 in the blood.[5] There's a more research supporting that.[6]

Interesting, isn't it? Let's get down to the prevention as well the cure of this rather simple issue that has seemed to have taken the best of us all. It is only public awareness on a massive scale that can prevent this disease from taking a hold of us, and this is what this book is for.

Chapter 2: The Basics

Bleeding Dogs and Vomit: The History of Vitamin B12
Until the 1920's, almost 6000 people all over the world lost their lives to pernicious anaemia – a disease that was characterised by severely low red blood cell counts, extreme lethargy, weakness and neuronal problems. The disease was said to be incurable back then and was believed to be due to some unidentified toxic substance in the blood due to which patients were offered treatments such as removal of their spleen, blood transfusions, etc. None of these treatments were working and it seemed that whoever got this disease had to die sooner or later.

With such a dismal state of affairs, most physicians were eagerly searching for the cure. In 1912, George Minot, a graduate of Harvard Medical School, started to believe that some particular substance present in food might be the cure for this disease. He had a keen interest in studying the diseases that affected the blood, maybe owing to the fact that Homer Wright (the developer of the staining techniques to prepare and study microscopic slides of blood) was one of his teachers. Consequently, Minot began the necessary investigations.

Minot was joined by William P. Murphy in 1923, also a graduate of Harvard Medical School. Together, they began to consider the work of George Whipple. Minot knew this researcher because they had worked together in Johns Hopkins together.

Whipple was also looking for a cure for pernicious anaemia and had been conducting experiments on dogs where he would bleed them to make them anaemic and then feed them different foods to see which types of foods cured their anaemia. He found out that liver was the best treatment and that red meat as well vegetables were helpful but to a lesser degree.

It wasn't long before Minot began to wonder if these findings could be of any use in humans. Murphy and Minot were both curious so they decided to find out by experimenting on their personal patients. They noticed that red blood cell counts were steadily increasing and therefore decided to try the administration of liver in hospitalised patients to find out if the treatment was really working.

As usually, when it comes to innovation (ask Steve Jobs), some of their colleagues were critical and some just didn't have faith in this experiment. However, Minot and Murphy did not follow Charles Hooper, another physician who had successfully treated 3 patients in 1918 by feeding them liver, only to desert his experiment later owing to the criticism and ridicule he faced from his colleagues and other physicians. Doctors simply couldn't believe that a disease as complex and distressing as pernicious anaemia could be due to a simple dietary deficiency.

Their will to never give up finally brought them success – the treatment initiated by Minot and Murphy worked. By 1926, they had treated 45 patients whose health had improved significantly within 2 weeks.

Whipple, Murphy and Minot were awarded the Nobel Prize in Physiology on December 12, 1934. In his banquet speech that day, Murphy said:

"We have been allowed the thrill of watching the patient through a few days of depression following the institution of liver therapy until remission occurs with its often sudden and almost unbelievable sense of well-being simultaneously with the maximum increase of the reticulocytes or new red blood cells. Then we have followed this remission through to completion, until the blood becomes normal, with a normal red blood cell level - that is 5,000,000 or more cells per cubic millimetre of blood. Perhaps even more dramatic has been the improvement in the disturbances of locomotion resulting from nerve damage."

That's one happy ending. But our story does not end here. Today we know that either a deficiency in the dietary intake of B12 or a problem in its metabolism within the body can account for its deficiency. Minot, Murphy and Whipple made the former very obvious, but how did we find out about the latter? We owe that to William Castle.

Up until Minot, Murphy and Whipple's work, no one knew what the liver contained that was the actual cure of pernicious anaemia. Castle, another Harvard graduate, had conducted numerous experiments to prove that a substance in the stomach had something to do with B12 deficiency. He had noticed that people who had their stomachs surgically removed commonly died due to pernicious anaemia even if meat or liver was fed to them. This meant that no matter how much of the cure was provided to them, there had to be another factor in the stomach which helped its uptake by the body.

To find out if this association was true, Castle dared to embark on one of the most gruesome experiments in the history of medical science. He ate meat, forcefully vomited it out and fed that vomitus to patients. As horrible as that sounds, it actually worked. That is to say that whatever was thrown out of his stomach had the potential to cure pernicious anaemia, just like liver or red meat. Castle called the substance within the body the 'intrinsic factor,' and that provided by the liver or meat the 'extrinsic factor.'

In 1948, the so-called 'extrinsic factor' was isolated and given the name of 'Vitamin B12'. Ever since that time, B12 has served to be the simple cure for the greatly disabling disease, pernicious anaemia. Inexpensive injections of B12 are one of the most favoured as well as inexpensive treatments for this disease today.

What is Vitamin B12

We've already discussed it quite briefly, but let's get a bit deeper into it. The term 'Vitamin B12' refers to a set of chemically related substances which are similar because all of them contain Cobalt, a rare metallic element. B12 is the largest and most complex of all the vitamins and is water-soluble.

The central Cobalt atom is held in the centre and different groups can be linked to it, each of them deciding the type of vitamin B12 that is finally made. For example, if the changeable group is cyanide, the final substance would be *cyanocobalamin*. Vitamin B12 refers to the following compounds (only two of which are used by the human body):

Cyanocobalamin: An inexpensive form of B12 that is easy to synthesise and is thus used widely as a food additive, in commercial preparations of B12, etc. It is made by purifying hydroxycobalamin along with using charcoal (which contains trace amounts of cyanide). In this reaction, cyanocobalamin is actually recovered as an artefact or an accidental, 'impure' substance.

Hydroxycobalamin: This contains a hydroxyl (-OH) group attached to the corrin ring, in addition to the unchangeable groups (the pyrrole rings). It is made by bacteria and is thus an expensive form, also used in medicines. It is expensive because it cannot be manufactured by a simple chemical reaction (as was cyanocobalamin) and we are solely dependent on bacteria for this form.

The two forms that the human body uses are the coenzymes **Adenosylcobalamin** and **Methylcobalamin**. Most enzymes of the human body are proteins by nature. A coenzyme is any non-protein substance that is absolutely necessary for certain enzymes to carry out their respective reactions.

The reactions that these enzymes take care of will be described when we get down to exploring the overall functions of B12 in the human body since it won't be fair to just state some complicated names of enzymes only to end up boring you.

*(**Note**: Bored? I feel you folks. If you wish to make more sense out of these facts, flip on to chapter 5, but don't forget to come back here once you're done.)*

Absorption of B12: The Major Pathway
Vitamin B12 is absorbed by a step-by-step process and a hindrance at any of these stages can cause problems in the uptake of vitamin B12. There are two pathways for this uptake:

Step 1
When you eat, B12 is bound to proteins in your diet. Within the saliva, the salivary glands also secrete certain binding proteins specific for B12. These are called R-binders or 'cobalophilins.' However, they do not bind to B12 within the oral cavity since it's already bound to proteins within the food. They travel with the food to the stomach.

Step 2

When you swallow, food carrying B12 enters your stomach, which releases a substance called 'pepsin' that helps remove the bond between proteins and B12, freeing it. As soon as the B12 is free, it binds to the R-binders that were secreted by the salivary glands. The stomach also produces 'intrinsic factor' which is another specific binding substance for B12 (yep, that vomit thingie). These 'binding factors' are important because B12 cannot be absorbed on its own, it needs to be associated with these proteins in order to be taken up by the gastrointestinal tract.

Step 3

Next, the B12 – R-binder complex enters the duodenum (the first part of your small intestine) and there, certain enzymes (which are released by your pancreas) break up this complex and B12 binds to the intrinsic factor that was secreted by your stomach.

Step 4

The B12-intrinsic factor complex enters the next part of the small intestine, i.e, the ileum, and B12 is taken up by the cells lining it.

Step 5

The cells of the ileum associate the B12 molecules with *transcobalamin*, a protein that helps carry B12 within the blood to all the organs that need it. These include the liver, the gastrointestinal tract's epithelium (the most superficial layer of the GIT), the bone marrow, etc.

Absorption of B12: The Minor Pathway

The pathway described above is the main route for the absorption of B12. However, another minor route also exists and deserves mention here since this is the pathway that serves to aid in B12 uptake when components of the major pathway are malfunctional or absent (such as in cases of stomach diseases, removal of the stomach, etc).

Sadly, the steps making up this route are not well-understood and all we know about it is the fact that it accounts for a very small percentage of the total absorption of B12 and that it does not depend on the ileum or the stomach for functioning properly.

So what's the importance of this alternative route? This alternative method of B12 absorption can help a person absorb around 1% of large oral doses in case he or she is suffering from B12 deficiency and cannot absorb it normally due to coexistent stomach diseases, intestinal malabsorption syndromes, etc. That's why people with B12 anaemia are given high oral doses of B12.

How Much B12 Do We Need Daily

Different age groups require varying amounts of B12. Most people consume foods that provide sufficient B12 (groups which are at risk of deficiency will be described next, in case you were wondering). Here are the recommended daily allowances of B12 for major age groups[7]:

0-6 months – 0.4 mcg
7-12 months – 0.5 mcg
1-3 years – 0.9 mcg
4-8 years – 1.2 mcg
9-13 years – 1.8 mcg
14+ years – 2.4 mcg

mcg stands for MICROgram. That's right, we're talking about very small amounts. Also, the recommended dose is the same for both men and women.

Dietary Requirements of B12 In Special Situations

In pregnant or lactating women, B12 is required in slightly higher amounts. The recommended daily allowance for pregnant women is 2.6 mcg and that for lactating mothers is 2.8 mcg[8], keeping in mind that the foetus or the baby needs the extra amount of B12 taken in.

What Is The Normal Range of B12 In The Body?

Now that you know how much B12 you need daily, let's look at how much B12 should be present in your blood to help your body function normally. Why do you need to know these? Well, it's not absolutely necessary for you to remember these since your doctor as well as your lab reports will usually point out whether your B12 levels are within the expected normal levels.

However, it's always better to be able to interpret your own lab results in order to understand any disease you might have. Although highly flawed and in urgent need of revision, the expected normal ranges of serum B12 that are commonly used are[9].

Newborn babies – 160-1300pg/ml
Adults – 200-900pg/ml
Breast milk – 180-300pg/ml

And here's how those ranges are interpreted:

<150 pg/ml = B12 deficiency
>200pg/ml = Adequate B12 levels
>900pg/ml = B12 excess (which doesn't cause any toxicity, therefore the term 'excess of B12' becomes rather spurious)

Caution: these values might be misleading! Here are a few things you need to know about them:

1. These ranges may vary slightly from one laboratory to another.

2. Different labs may use different units for the expression of B12 levels in the serum.

3. Most labs have set the standard values somewhat too low[10] since many people have been reported to be suffering from the symptoms of B12 deficiency even though their serum B12 was within normal limits.[11] There's more[12] and more research validating that[13], Therefore, if you get a lab test and continue to suffer from the symptoms of B12 deficiency, it might be time for you to consult a different doctor or even a B12 specialist.

4. Do not ignore your symptoms since this disease can lead to catastrophic consequences (even though it is extremely easy and inexpensive to treat) only because it remains undiagnosed in many people. These ranges are definitely 'too low' and many people have symptoms at the so-called adequate ranges. Don't forget this!

To know about what the acceptable values SHOULD be, refer to Chapter 4.

Where Do We Get Our B12 From

The importance of this question cannot be overemphasised. All people who are at risk of developing B12 deficiency should know which foods are the best sources of B12 [14]since consuming natural food products is always better than mere medications or supplements. Let's look at the sources of vitamin B12 first and then discuss why it might be better to consume these foods as compared to getting supplements or B12 injections.

The general principle, as I mentioned earlier in the introductory chapter, is that bacteria make B12 and these bacteria are present in the gastrointestinal tracts of animals which is why animal sources are the best sources of B12 and that present in vegetables is only because of contamination. Otherwise, plants have literally no B12 within them.

When talking about sources, it's always handy to classify them into natural, synthetic and fortified ones. The synthetic ones include oral supplements or vitamin b12 injections, something which forms the bulk of B12 deficiency treatment in individuals who cannot consume B12 via natural food sources owing to the fact that they are either strict vegetarians or have some disease or condition (such as sprue, auto immune gastritis, gastrectomy) which does not allow effective B12 uptake. It's important that we go through the natural sources before considering the man-made alternatives

Natural-Food Sources:

Overall, shellfish and animal products (meat and poultry) are believed to contain the highest amount of Vitamin B12.

Seafood

Shellfish contains large amounts of B12 and some of them are great sources of other elemental nutrients such as Iron, Zinc and Potassium.

Clams are the richest source of B12, providing 99 µg in just 100g. In addition, clams are also the richest source of iron and provide considerable amounts of potassium as well.

Oysters also supply iron along with the B12, the latter being present in amounts varying from 16-17 µg in six medium-sized oysters. However, make sure you buy the farmed Pacific ones since the wild ones are usually contaminated.

Next in line is **Caviar or fish eggs,** which are mostly used as a spread in various dishes. 56.4 µg of vitamin B12 is present in 100 g of eggs of whitefish. Caviar (eggs of the Sturgeon fish) contains about 20 µg of B12 per 100 g.

Octopus contains 36 µg of B12 in the cooked state and 20 µg per 100 grams in the raw state. Various types of fish also provide B12, with the highest amount of B12 being present in **Mackerel**, which supplies 19 µg per 100 gram serving. This is followed by Herring, Salmon, Tuna, etc.

When it comes to **Crabs and Lobsters**, 11.5 µg of B12 are present in every 100 grams of Crabs and 4.04 µg of B12 in every 100 grams of Lobsters.

Land Animals

Beef liver contains around 83µg of vitamin B12 every 100 grams, **Turkey liver** contains about 43µg of B12 per 100g, whereas simmered **chicken liver** gives around 20µg per 100g. **Lamb or Mutton** gives 3.71µg/100g from the shoulder. The fore shank, leg and lamb chops provide successively lesser amounts of B12. In addition to B12, Beef provides heme-iron, protein and zinc whereas Lamb is a good source of protein and zinc.

As you see, **Liver** is the best source of B12 when it comes to land-animal derived foods. The largest amount of B12 is provided by the liver of lamb, followed by veal, moose, turkey, duck and goose. Lamb liver contains 85.7 µg per 100 grams serving. Kidneys and some other internal organs also contain an impressive amount of B12.

Cheese provides varying amounts of B12 depending on what type it is with the largest amount being supplied by Swiss cheese, which gives about 3.34 µg per 100 grams. Cheese is also a good source of proteins, vitamin B2 and calcium. The same principle also applies to **eggs**, i.e, the type decides the amount of B12 available in it. Chicken eggs contain most of the B12 in the raw yellow, giving 1.95 µg per 100 g serving, or

19

0.33 µg per egg.

Note From Regev: Always opt to buy only grass-fed, pasture-raised free-cage organic animals. Not only are they more ethically raised (to me, at least), but are also much healthier. They contain no fertilisers, chemicals, antibiotics and other bad stuff. A word of caution has to be said about dairy as well. Consume it only if you seem to tolerate it, and even then - make sure they are from pasture-raised, grass-fed free-roaming cows. Don't be afraid of the fats if they're properly raised. The major problem is lactose (dairy sugar) and if you buy full-fat fermented dairy (yoghurt, kefir, cheese) – lactose is mostly gone due to the fermentation.

Fortified Cereals?

Although certain types of cereals are fortified with B12, it's not wise to rely on these. Grains are also a troublesome piece of food (which is what cereals are made of), but it is way beyond the scope of this book. If you're a vegetarian, you have a lot better choices. Keep reading on.

Supplemental Sources

These include B12 supplements and injections. However, before moving on to this form of B12, it's necessary we discuss the disease manifestations of B12 and how it causes these to understand the various treatment options for those suffering from B12 deficiency or those at risk of developing it.

Myths About Special B12-Rich Foods For Vegans

After finding some papers stating the values of vegan foods with respect to B12, I went to 'interrogate' a professor of medicine whom I greatly admire and trust. The subject of the matter was soy products, yeast extracts, margarine and other vegan - so-called - sources of B12.

He appeared to be in deep thought when suddenly; he picked up his phone and began chatting away with some friend of his. He handed the phone to me, saying 'Here's an old classmate and friend of mine, she's a nutritionist. I give you my word that she is a very reliable and knowledgeable person.'

(She chose to stay anonymous, so let's simply refer to her as A.S)

When I curiously asked her if she agrees with the common assumption that vegans can rely on fortified cereals, soy products, yeast extracts and some margarines for keeping their B12 levels high enough, she replied:

> **Dr. A.S:** *Absolutely not! Only a few fortified cereals that have good amounts of B12 are available in the market. The rest of the sources are not useful at all – there's a lot of controversy about yeast extracts but there's literally no B12 in soy products.*

My colleagues were mentioning some research papers stating that soy products do contain B12. Why are those sources stating such facts?

> **Dr. A.S:** *Well, I can't say as to why they're stating such facts but here's the thing: Do not believe in just about anything that you read online. In addition, there's so many of them that we usually cannot decide which one to follow since many make contradicting statements.*
>
> *Therefore, don't follow these blogs/websites/magazines unless you're extremely certain that the writer is a qualified, experienced person – the eventual diagnosis and diet suggestions coming from your doctor and nutritionist.*
>
> *Personally, I rely on the data provided by the USDA (United States Department of Agriculture) for individuals residing in the west since it's different for different regions of the world. You can go to their website and download the list that states the amount of B12 in different foods directly from there.*

(Here's the link, in case you're interested. This page lists all the nutrients, you can scroll down and find B12 and download its associated data).

Chit-chatting about the efficiency and reliability of these sources for vegans, she expressly exclaimed:

> **Dr. A.S:** *No, I wouldn't recommend them at all. You can take*

fortified cereals in small amounts but that's definitely not enough. Why rely on these controversial sources when you have the widely accepted and easy-to-use supplements? I recommend that all vegans, whether they are consuming fortified cereals or not, should take these supplements. That will make sure they always have the required amounts of B12 in their body.

If you're curious enough for a reliable source for looking up the reference intakes for various nutrients, Dr. A.S got you on this one as well! She recommends this source.

To sum up, this means **there are no reliable vegan sources of B12**[15] **and no vegetarian should live without regular B12 supplementation**[16]. **Even 'The Vegan Society'** [17] **supports this!**[18]

Why Do People Develop B12 Deficiency

If I were to read about something that described how deficiencies develop and what symptoms they cause, I would look for information regarding who could develop the deficiency and why. The symptoms would be easier to understand once I had all that background information.

Keeping that in mind, I've tried listing most of the groups of individuals or the types of conditions that can lead to this deficiency. Before you go through that, let's recall a few basic points and add in a little more to understand the next section (which deals with the high-risk groups) better. Here you go:

B12 is absorbed via a number of steps which involve the R-Binder from the saliva, the intrinsic factor from the stomach and finally *transcobalamin-II* in the ileum (after getting absorbed here) to be delivered to the organs that need it. A problem at any of these steps can lead to impairment of B12 absorption, even if you are taking in enough B12 in your food.

B12 associates with toxins and helps in their removal from your body, getting excreted with them eventually. That means too many toxins in your body (for example alcohol or tobacco) can reduce the amount of B12 in your body.

B12 is stored in large amounts in your body and its deficiency can take years to show up because the body will use its available stores of this vitamin to counter the state of deficiency.

B12 deficiency is more commonly associated with faulty absorption of the vitamin as opposed to low intake of the vitamin itself.

Keeping the above in mind, let's explore the high-risk groups for B12 deficiency along with looking for the causes of their association with this condition:

Group A: People With a Low B12 Intake

1. Vegetarians.

2. Infants of vegetarian mothers (who are being breast fed by them[19] and are not given dairy products or fortified formula milk).[20]

3. Underprivileged people who simply cannot afford to eat a healthy diet that constitutes of enough B12-rich animal foods (common in the third world countries).

4. People who have chronic disorders which do not allow them to take in adequate amounts of B12, or any type of food for that matter, such as *Anorexia Nervosa* (a psychiatric condition which makes a patient perceive himself as overweight and makes him/her starve himself even when he might be grossly underweight), *Bulimia* (also a psychiatric condition due to which patients eat large or fatty meals and force themselves to vomit out whatever they eat in order to stay thin), and more.

Group B: People With a Normal B12 Intake But an Impaired Absorption

If you have the basics of absorption in mind, this part shouldn't be hard to guess. Of course, the removal or malfunctioning of any of the involved organs in the step-by-step absorption of B12 can cause a state of severe B12 deficiency even when the patient is consuming large amounts of B12 in his/her diet. Here are the associated conditions/diseases:

*Problems arising in the **stomach***:

The stomach produces intrinsic factor, a protein that allows B12 to be absorbed into the ileum. Parietal cells produce this substance and any damage to them can result in B12 deficiency. Below are the associated major subgroups:

Conditions that cause parietal cell dysfunction include atrophic gastritis (a disease in which the immune system of the body mistakenly attacks the gastric parietal cells, destroying them completely, leading to a disease called pernicious anaemia) and *H.Pylori Gastritis* (a very common infection of the stomach that in some individuals, damages the parietal cells and leads to atrophic gastritis, thus reducing intrinsic factor and B12 absorption. It is easily treatable by antibiotics).

Conditions that cause loss of the stomach[21] include those diseases in which the whole stomach or parts of it have to be removed[22]. These obviously include cancers of the stomach itself, oesophageal cancer which has spread to and invaded some part of the stomach, stomach surgery for weight loss which results in the loss of a part of the stomach.[23]

(many a time, this is the part that contains the parietal cells and thus, the remaining part of the stomach cannot produce intrinsic factor for B12 absorption).

Conditions that lower acid production in the stomach cause B12 deficiency because acid is required to break up the bond within the B12-Protien complex since B12 is bound to proteins within your food and is not just 'floating around' freely.

Diseases that lower acid production include *achlorhydria* (absence of the production of acid in the stomach, which can be due to autoimmune gastritis), Gastric bypass surgery, the combined Antrectomy plus Vagotomy procedure (an out-dated surgical procedure designed to reduce the amount of acid production by the stomach) and a rare genetic disorder called *Mucolipidosis type IV*.

*Problems arising in the **pancreas**:*

You might recall that the pancreas release the enzyme which frees the B12 from the B12 - R-binder complex, if this enzyme is absent or decreased in amount, B12 will not be removed from that complex and won't be absorbed. The conditions that can cause such a situation are:

Decreased amount of the protease that frees B12 from the B12 – R-binder complex: Anything that causes pancreatic insufficiency can cause this, such as cystic fibrosis, chronic alcoholism, pancreatic cancer, etc.

Inactivation of the enzymes released by the pancreas: This can occur if there is too much acid, something that occurs in *Zollinger-Ellison* syndrome.

*Problems arising in the **small intestine**:*

If you recall your basics, the intestine is the part where the intrinsic factor-B12 complex is absorbed; B12 is freed and attached to *Transcobalamin-II* to be circulated in the blood *for utilisation by vario*us organs.

Anything going wrong in the ileum (a part of the small intestine responsible for B12 absorption) can cause a B12 deficiency. Let's have a look at the conditions that can cause problems in the ileum:

General malabsorption syndromes of the gastrointestinal tract which impair the uptake of all nutrients, including B12.

Celiac Disease (in which the lining of the ileum is damaged and cannot take up B12).

Crohn's disease (a disease in which the immune system attacks the gastrointestinal tract, affecting literally any part of the GIT. When the small intestine is involved, malabsorption can occur).

Surgical removal of the ileum (this occurs in people who have cancer of the intestines whether primary or secondary, and in those who have had their ileum removed due to uncontrollable Crohn's disease).

Group C: People with Both Normal Intake and Absorption of B12

If you read the above title twice, don't worry – anyone, including myself, would do the same. It definitely sounds absurd. Here are the conditions which hinder the utilization and/or absorption of vitamin B12 in the body even when all the organs needed for absorption are normal and intake is enough to meet the daily requirements:

Chronic infestations by parasites (mainly worms) that reside in the human intestine and take up many nutrients from the food taken in. Fish tapeworm, found around Canada and Alaska, competes with the gut for absorption of B12, causing its deficiency. According to some studies, another parasitic infection of the GIT, called *Giardiasis*, also causes B12 deficiency.[24]

Overgrowth of the normally present bacteria in the gut also leads to B12 deficiency since these little creatures start eating up the B12 meant for your own organs.

Bacterial overgrowth is not an actual disease; it is just a consequence of conditions of the gut which favour the stasis and growth of bacteria, the prime example of such a disease being *diverticulosis*.

In this condition, sac-like dilatations form in the gut and bacteria start accumulating here, their large numbers affecting the nutrient amounts available for your own body.

Group D: People Taking Drugs That Interact With B12[25]

Some medications and toxins interact with B12 and decrease its levels in the serum[26], either by inhibiting its uptake or causing a greater excretion. The following list summarises most of such substances[27]:

Metformin, a drug used widely for the treatment and management of Diabetes Mellitus as well as Polycystic Ovary Disease in women, lowers B12 uptake in the gastrointestinal tract. According to reports, many of the patients (approximately 30%) who have been taking this drug for a long time period develop a B12 deficiency[28]. There's a LOT of further scientific validation[29] for it.[30] The relation of Metformin to a B12 deficiency is well documented[31]. So if you're a diabetic or have polycystic ovary disease, consult your doctor about B12 supplementation if you're taking Metformin.

Drugs that lower acidity of the stomach[32] (Proton Pump Inhibitors and H^2 Receptor Blockers) also decrease B12 absorption from food (but not from supplements since this form of B12 is not bound to proteins and thus does not require acid to be separated from the complex).

People who have gastrointestinal reflux disease, peptic ulcers or acidity are on chronic therapy that includes these drugs and thus need to be given supplemental B12 while they are on treatment. This doesn't mean that if you take these drugs for a few months, you're going to end up with a B12 deficiency.

Some reports indicate you'd have to take H^2 Receptor Blockers for at least 2 years, etc – the overall deductions being somewhat contradictory.[33] However, one thing we can all agree on is that long-term therapy with these drugs needs to be monitored[34], very carefully[35]. More[36] and more[37] studies[38] confirm that.

Alcohol is a toxin and B12 removes toxins from the body[39], as explained earlier. Chronic alcoholism significantly reduces B12 levels in the blood and thus, alcoholics need to reduce alcohol intake and/or B12 supplementation regularly.

Those who take *salicylates* (Aspirin) for long periods, such as patients of heart disease, can develop B12 deficiency. Similarly, the anti-tuberculosis drug *Isoniazid*, which is chemically similar to the salicylates, cause a similar situation, necessitating the concurrent therapy of B12 supplements.

Some **antibiotics** interact with B12 by decreasing its ability to make up new red blood cells, provided that both the antibiotic and B12 are given together. This does not mean that anyone who has an infection will develop a B12 deficiency if he or she is given one of these antibiotics, it only applies to those people who are already deficient in B12. In simple terms, anyone who is being given B12 for the treatment of a deficiency should not be given certain antibiotics (those belonging to the **amino-glycoside** group, such as gentamicin, tobramycin, etc) because these decrease the efficacy of B12.

Drugs used for the treatment of epilepsy, such as *phenobarbital*, *pheytoin* and *primidone* are associated with low B12 levels in the serum.

Zidovudine, an anti-viral drug used for the management of AIDS, decreases B12 levels in the blood and B12 supplementation in these patients is necessary.

Colchicine, a drug used to treat gout, also lowers B12 levels.

Group E: People With Increased B12 Needs

(Could you be one of them?)

Without further ado, let's get practical and look at which age groups are at the highest risk of developing B12 deficiency so that we can finally move on towards the signs of deficiency (phew!):

Elderly Individuals[40]: This age group is at risk[41] because of the observation that around 20-30 percent (different studies state different percentages) of people above the age of 50 years develop atrophic gastritis, a disease which directly reduces B12 absorption[42] as described earlier. Numerous studies[43] confirm that[44].

Children: Children do not have adequate stores of B12 as compared to adults so low intake or malabsorption in case of a child could result in a

B12 deficiency considerably well before it would in an adult.

Pregnant females/lactating mothers: Since the fetus or the breast-fed child draws out nutrients from his/her mother's body, it is obvious that the mother can develop a deficiency of just about any nutrient if she is not taking in the extra amount that is being delivered to her baby through her.

Those who have gastrointestinal surgery: As explained earlier, if you have had any surgery due to which a part of your stomach or ileum was removed, you will need much more B12 than other people.

Group F: People with Genetic Problems

The genes responsible for B12 metabolism might be affected due to which absorption or usage of this vitamin could be affected – eight such genes have been identified so far (June, 2012).

For Geeks Only: What is Zollinger-Ellison syndrome?

This is a condition which is classically made of a triad of three symptoms: increased amounts of acid in the stomach, peptic ulcers and a non-beta cell tumour of the pancreas (gastrinoma).

The excessive acid inactivates the pancreatic enzymes which are necessary to free B12 from the R-binders. Patients who have this syndrome have abdominal pain and diarrhoea.

It is usually due to a tumour or ectopic gastric tissue present anywhere in the GIT (commonly pancreas and the duodenum) which releases gastrin, the hormone that stimulates acid production. The excessive acid causes ulceration as well as inactivation of the pancreatic enzymes.

The Signs & Symptoms of B12 Deficiency

Vitamin B12 deficiency presents with a wide range of signs and symptoms[45], the most common ones being those related to anaemia and neuropathy (damage to or alteration of the normal functioning of nerves). Low levels of vitamin B12 affect all the systems of the body, as shows below:

The Gastrointestinal Tract: Bloating, indigestion, constipation, diarrhoea, Abdominal discomfort or pain, oral ulcers, gingival bleeding (bleeding from the gums), loss of appetite, weight loss, thickening of the tongue and malabsorption.

The Cardiovascular System: Chest pain, heart attacks, stroke, increased heart rate, deep venous thrombosis (a condition in which clots form in the veins of the legs, causing pain and putting the patient at risk of dying suddenly due to breakage of these clots and transfer to the blood vessels of the lung, blocking them in turn and causing respiratory failure) and enlargement of the heart.

The Nervous System: Altered sensations, depression, psychosis, mania, confusion, fatigue, suicidal thought, anger, phobias, apathy, irritability, delusions, hallucinations, loss of memory, exaggerated reflexes, tremors, cramps, numbness, pins and needles sensations and paralysis.

The Immune System: Impairment of the immune system in a way that lowers its ability to fight infections and heal wounds efficiently.

Ear, Nose and Throat: Dizziness, vertigo (when the patient feels that his/her surroundings are spinning around him), imbalance, hearing problems and difficulty in swallowing.

Eyes: Blindness, double vision, tunnel vision, nystagmus (abnormal movements of the eye which do not correspond with the movements of the head) and pain in or at the back of the eye.

The Respiratory System: Asthma, shortness of breath and wheezing.

The Genitourinary System: Incontinence, decreased libido, increased urinary tract infections, infertility, menstrual problems and impotence.

The Endocrine System: Hypothyroidism (which presents with fatigue, weight gain, muscle pain, low blood pressure and depression), infertility and diabetes.

The Haematological System (Blood and blood-cells): Anaemia, increased infections and faulty wound healing, fatigue and breathlessness.

The Musculoskeletal System: Increased risk of fractures in the elderly population, muscular spasms and cramps, chronic severe muscular pain and fatigue, osteoporosis (weakening of the bones) and bone pain.

Dermatological manifestations: Dry skin, brittle nails, dry and lifeless hair, increased hair fall and early onset of the greying of hair.

Stages of B12 Deficiency

Above we listed all the possible symptoms that can arise due to a B12 deficiency. However, most of those who suffer from this condition will present with just a few or a handful number of these symptoms, the exact order being completely unpredictable.

Although B12 deficiency does not follow a regular pattern, let's look at its stages (which have been devised only for convenience since the exact pattern of the symptomology depends on various factors such as genetics, dietary habits, etc) before moving on to the detailed description of each system affected by it and how exactly it does so:

Stage 1:

This is just the beginning of the deficiency and is only represented by low serum B12 levels. It has absolutely no signs or symptoms.

Stage 2:

In this stage, the levels of B12 are not only low in the serum but are also decreased within the cells, therefore cellular dysfunction sets in. Symptoms are usually not present in this stage.

Stage 3:

In this stage, the levels of *methylmalonic acid* and *homocysteine* are both increased in the blood. Don't worry, as hard as those names sound, the concept is pretty simple. B12 is involved in reactions which convert these substances to other forms to complete certain functions in the body (such as DNA synthesis).

When B12 is not available, these substances can no longer be converted in to the form the body needs, thus their levels begin to rise. That's pretty much it as far as the chemical stuff goes. What about the symptoms? Patients at this stage of the disease experience neurological, psychological as well as mild gastrointestinal symptoms.

These include lethargy, weakness, confusion, decreased attention span, numbness and mild tingling sensations, abdominal discomfort, indigestion, mild diarrhoea and bloating. However, this stage characteristically does not have anaemia, a feature of the last stage of B12 deficiency.

Stage 4:

This is the final and most severe stage of B12 deficiency and without prompt treatment, the nervous system of such patients can be damaged permanently. That means that if you don't get treated on time, you might get irreversible brain damage (which could be dubbed as Alzheimer's) or complete paralysis of a part of your body owing damage to the nerve that supplies that region

That's just the facts, I'm not trying to scare you. Be careful about what you decide when it comes to getting diagnosed and treated for this deficiency – it is most definitely NOT to be taken lightly. In addition, anaemia is usually apparent at this stage and causes severe lethargy, pallor, weakness and breathlessness.

The Most Dangerous Symptoms of B12 Deficiency
Even the slightest dysfunction in the human body can cause a person a great discomfort and disrupt his daily activities. Those symptoms that are treatable are obviously not considered dangerous.

However, certain conditions produce permanent impairments if not treated on time and B12 deficiency is definitely one of them. The nervous system does not have the ability to regenerate itself once it is damaged and sadly, the 'safe window' of this particular system is very narrow.

That means that very little damage or constant insult to this system for a short time period can result in irreparable harm, giving us a very a short time to diagnose and treat the cause before it gets too late. B12 damages the nervous system directly and if stage 3 and 4 are not treated immediately, irreversible damage occurs to the nervous system, symptoms of which include:

1, Severe mental dysfunction (which can range from psychosis to mania or even hallucinations).

2. Memory loss

3. Paralysis

4. Blindness

5. Tunnel Vision (explained in detail in the section on how B12 deficiency affects the eyes).

6. Permanent alteration of sensations in the limbs (Parasthesias).

7. Bladder and bowel incontinence.

Once these symptoms set in, no matter how well you get treated, the normal functions of the nervous system will not return. So, before it gets too late, get a screening test and consult your doctor.

If you think anyone around you might have the symptoms of a B12 deficiency, advise them to see a doctor and get the necessary tests done. After all, it's just a few tests, right? A tiny bit of effort could save you and your loved ones from these severe and crippling symptoms.

Chapter 3: Putting It All Together

B12's Functions and How Its Deficiency Can Affect You
Functions of B12[46]

By now, you know that B12 deficiency can affect just about any organ of the body. But how? The fresh medical student might think: 'Hey, it's used in just 2 chemical reactions in the body, how come it affects all organ systems?' If a medical student has crossed his/her first year of education, they will probably think 'Okay, most organ systems can be affected, but how come all of them are listed as being involved in this book?'

Then, you folks out there who have nothing to do with the medical profession and are keen readers very concerned about their health will most definitely be overwhelmed by these facts and might even think of giving this whole business a rest. You should neither be sceptical or overwhelmed – don't just put this book down yet. You still haven't learnt the most beautiful thing about vitamin B12's role in the body. Once you know that, you'll get the why and how it affects so many organs, mostly multiple organs at the same time.

1. Involvement in DNA Synthesis – *B12's most interesting and important function*

The simplest thing that you should never forget about B12 is that it is necessary for the formation of DNA – the genetic material in almost all the cells of the body.

It makes DNA – then what? This simply signifies the fact that those cells that are dividing fast will be affected the most because the more they divide, the greater the amount of DNA synthesis since each new cell that stems from its parent cell (recalling our biology basics now, aren't we?) will need its own DNA, which obviously has to be manufactured sometime before the cell divides.

The cells of the gastrointestinal tract, bone marrow and skin belong to the most rapidly dividing group of cells in the body. I'll tell you more when each of these systems are discussed in further details, let's just go through everything step-by-step.

2. Synthesis of Red Blood Cells – *folate's trapped, B12 to the rescue!*

Here's the thing: Folate is required for the synthesis of red blood cells, those tiny disc-shaped cells that carry oxygen in your blood to deliver it to each and every corner of your body. However, B12 is required in a reaction that converts folate into a form usable by the body to make red blood cells. Without that, folate cannot participate in the synthesis of red blood cells. So without B12, folate is literally of no use![47]

3. Tingling, Pins & Needles, Numbness – *B12's connection to a myriad of funny sensations which aren't funny at all*

Vitamin B12 is required for the normal functioning of the nervous system because it is essential for the synthesis and repair of a protective sheath wrapped around every nerve fibre in your body – the myelin sheath.

Without this layer, the nerves cannot transmit their impulses and if they stay completely stripped off of the myelin sheath, they eventually die.

That's why people with a B12 deficiency develop abnormal sensations[48], altered gaits (ataxia), etc. Don't worry; you'll hear more on this interesting topic once we get down to the nervous system.

4. Feeling a little low? Try a shot of B12! *B12 Deficiency & Depression* [49]

Well, not literally! You would obviously have to get certain tests before your B12 supplementation can be justified. B12 is involved in the metabolism of a chemical called "Homocysteine," a substance that is associated with depression, schizophrenia, Alzheimer's disease[50] and non-specific mood disorders.

That's because without B12, homocysteine is not converted into the form the body needs[51] and it begins to accumulate in the blood, damaging the nervous system as well as the heart (which is why it is associated with cardiovascular disease, described later).

Further research[52] confirms that[53].

5. No B12? No Energy! *B12 and energy production*

Vitamin B12 is involved in the conversion of carbohydrates and fats into ATP – the energy currency of your body. Without it, these substances cannot be utilised well and you won't be getting the energy you wish to derive from the food you eat. So remember, all that yummy food won't be of any benefit if there isn't enough B12 in your body.

6. Hormones and B12 – *B12's effects on the endocrine system*

The hormones in your body serve numerous important functions and need a fully functional cell membrane – something that surrounds each and every cell of your body. Without a healthy cell membrane, hormones cannot enter the cells in your body to produce the effects they are normally supposed to produce. That's because these chemicals need special receptors to get inside your cells. Since these receptors are present on the cell membranes, damage to the cell membranes makes the receptors unstable, making it impossible for the hormones to get into the cells of your body. Thus, without B12's stabilising effect on your cell membranes, most of your hormones will just float around in your blood till they're excreted. What a sad, sad fate.

7. Your Own Body Trying to Destroy Its Organs – *B12's connection to auto-immune diseases*

Auto-immune diseases comprise a fairly large group of conditions in which the body's immune system faultily recognises the body's own components as 'foreign' and launches an immune attack on them. Under normal conditions, there are special substances attached to each and every cell of your body which are sort of like 'markers,' telling the cells of your immune system, 'You're completely unauthorised to attack me, I'm a national of this state.'

These markers are attached to your cell membrane and like I said earlier, B12 is one of the factors that contribute to the stability of the cell membranes. Once they are faulty, those markers will fall off and your own immune cells will fail to recognise the rest of the cells of your body, attacking them, 'thinking' they're foreign invaders.

For Geeks Only: What reactions in the human body use vitamin B12?

The enzyme methionine synthase uses B12 (in the form of methylcobalamin) to convert homocysteine to methionine. In this reaction, methylcobalamin serves as a cofactor.

The enzyme methylmalonyl-coenzyme A mutase uses B12 (in the form of adenosylcobalamin, a prosthetic group in this case) to isomerize methylmalonyl coenzyme A to succinyl coenzyme A.

B12 Deficiency & Anaemia
When Red Blood Cells Are Born Too Early and Die Too Soon

Have you ever had the chance to see a child who is weak, malnourished and has been diagnosed to have anaemia? Most of you probably haven't. I've seen pregnant women who are slightly anaemic, I've seen patients with *tuberculosis* who are on medications and become anaemic and weak – but none of them were as bad as seeing a 2 year old child appear as if he were only 6 months old.

His skin was dry, his hair was scarce, and he had been getting various types of infections due to his bad health. His was a premature birth – he was 28 weeks old when he was delivered. Of course, the medical student will be listing all the causes of that in his head and the doctor will be thinking of the possible complica.. (disk scratch)

Stop right there. Just take a moment and imagine if a child close to you looked like that – all due to something as simple as the deficiency of a nutrient which wasn't letting him grow and develop normally. Would you let that happen to your child? Would you let something destroy his/her health when you could prevent it or treat it fairly easily? Of course you wouldn't.

Although this child's state was far too suggestive of an anaemia, your child might not be so easily diagnosed because early symptoms are not easily noticeable, especially in children who cannot tell you that they are tired or feeling low.

Not only children, but even adults can go unnoticed. That's why this deficiency has most rightly been called a 'silent epidemic' by many people. B12 won't present with severe symptoms in the beginning – children are at even more danger because they don't have stores of this vitamin, like adults often do.

What's worse is that they might not even be able to tell you what's wrong with them. Observe your children closely and do not make any delays in taking them to the doctor. Don't forget that it is you who has to take the first step – it is you who reports to the doctor first, no physician will come to you himself. Take your first step and don't give up. Keep a close watch on yourself and your loved ones and spread the word amongst those who do not know- we must fight this battle together.

The Background

Prematurity is a risk factor for multiple complications, whether you talk about a premature birth or a premature decision regarding an important milestone in your life. Likewise, all the cells in your body go through various stages of development to achieve their mature status which is their fully functional form. If they do not mature on time and are 'released' to do their work, they won't obviously be able to carry it out too well.

That's what happens to your red blood cells when you develop a B12 deficiency. Your red blood cells are usually derived from already existing 'stem cells' within your bone marrow – a soft, spongy and fleshy area within some of your bones that eventually gives rise to all the cells within your blood such as red blood cells (the ones that carry oxygen), white blood cells (the ones that fight infection) and platelets (the ones that make you clot when you bleed).

All these cells produced by the marrow have varying life spans and need to be replaced after a certain period of time, which means that the marrow has to keep functioning almost at a constant rate and its metabolic needs as well as cellular growth rate are both high.

Before a cell divides, it enters a phase where it synthesises extra DNA and other necessary substances which have to be transferred to the new cell which will arise from it after it divides in two. The more these cells divide, the greater the amount of DNA that they need. Although mature red blood cells do not contain DNA, their younger stages do. Without fully functional DNA, cells cannot work since the DNA contains all the genes which direct the activities of the cell, ranging from various enzymes to receptors and the likes (in addition to deciding what your eye colour is and how tall you will be).

So now you know that rapidly dividing cells need more DNA and without healthy DNA, they will be malfunctional, but where does B12 fit in? That's the best part of this intricate story.

For DNA synthesis, two vitamins are required : vitamin B12 and vitamin B9 (Folic Acid). Vitamin B12 is used by an enzyme that converts Vitamin B9 into a form usable by the body to make DNA. Therefore, when you don't have enough B12 in your body, all the folic acid in your diet will be useless and your bone marrow will not be able to use it to make DNA for the huge number of cells it has to grow, nourish and release into your blood once they are mature.

So, no B12 means no folic acid. That leads to faulty cell production in the marrow. What happens next? Well, your bone marrow will still try to make red blood cells but these will not be mature since their DNA is what directs all the activities which lead them to acquire maturity. In the marrow, immature cells are large and flimsy whereas mature cells have a smaller, more rigid shape.

Red blood cells have a disc-like shape. When they're immature, they will look large and their cell membranes will be flimsy, something that makes their life shorter than that of a normal red blood cell. That is because red blood cells have to travel through very narrow spaces (such as the sinusoids in the spleen) and their special cell membrane lets them squeeze through.

However, this won't be possible with the malfunctional cell membrane, thus putting these red blood cells at risk of getting damaged and broken down when they have to pass through tiny spaces. That's why they'll end up dying earlier. A premature birth and an early death, a sad ending indeed for these tiny fellows who could have lived a normal life only if you had fed your marrow some B12.

One More Look at the Signs and Symptoms

Your red blood cells carry oxygen, the basic requirement of all your tissues for survival. Without it, your cells grow weak and weary because they won't be able to generate energy for carrying out their basic functions. The concept is pretty simple. The signs and symptoms aren't that hard to get either. Let's suppose that you don't consume enough B12 and develop Anaemia (low red blood cell count or low haemoglobin, the red pigment in your RBCs that carries oxygen and makes your blood red). Here's what you could experience or feel:

Pale and dull skin (since the red/pink colour is imparted by haemoglobin within your RBCs, which are now unhealthy and dying too early).

Increased heart rate (Your heart can sense, albeit indirectly, that your tissues are not getting enough oxygen. This makes it pump faster to compensate for the low blood supply/oxygen delivery to the tissues).

Palpitations (this means that you will be aware of your own heartbeat).

Weakness and a feeling of general malaise, tiredness, etc (owing to the fact that your tissues are not getting enough oxygen and just a little work depletes them of all their energy stores).

Diarrhoea

Sore tongue and cracks at the corners of the mouth

If your anaemia is severe and prolonged, you might start experiencing constricting chest pain (angina) and sharp pain in your legs when you walk (something tat doctors call intermittent claudication).

In severe cases, headaches can also occur.

Additional symptoms include hair loss and eczema-like skin problems

However, if your child has anaemia, they might not be able to tell about what they feel which is why you should look out for signs of:

Pale skin

Irritability

Laziness/weakness

Low concentration span

Diarrhoea

Failure to eat/drink properly (babies with anaemia will not be able to take in milk or any semi-solid food that you give them simply because they don't have the energy to do it).

Red, swollen tongue

Cracks at the angles of the mouth (something doctors like to call 'angular stomatitis').

Thin nails

Drowsiness

Sore tongue

For Geeks Only: What is Addison's Anaemia?

Addison's Anaemia, Biermer's anaemia and Addison–Biermer anaemia are all different terms used to refer to Pernicious Anaemia.

B12 Deficiency Anaemia, on the other hand, is also sometimes referred to as Megaloblastic Anaemia since it is one of the causes of enlarged red blood cells, the other cause being Folic Acid Deficiency.

'Megaloblast' means an abnormally large red blood cell that contains DNA, a feature not present in mature RBCs.

What is Pernicious Anaemia

Although there are multiple causes of B12 deficiency, as I described earlier in the causes section, this particular condition deserves a separate explanation.

Pernicious Anaemia affects a large number of individuals and is an auto-immune disorder. Yes, that means that the body attacks its own cells. In this case, the immune system attacks and destroys the cells of the stomach that produce intrinsic factor, the substance necessary for B12's absorption in the ileum.

Without that, no B12 is absorbed and these patients develop a severe

B12 deficiency which needs regular and life-long B12 supplementation.

For Geeks Only: What is Myelosis Funicularis?

This is the name given to the complex of symptoms that are associated with neurological abnormalities due to B12 deficiency:

Altered perception of pressure, vibration, touch, constant and frustrating parasthesias.

Decreased or absent deep muscle-tendon reflexes.

Dorsal Cord Ataxia.

Abnormal reflexes such as Babinski response, etc.

Paralysis.

B12 and the Nervous System

There are tens of thousands of genes intricately folded up to form your DNA, the ultra-small structure that decides what you look like, what colour your hair will be and even how long you will live.

Our immune systems are designed to attack anything that is foreign and gain entry into our body. However, nature has proposed a mechanism that stops a mother's body from attacking the foetus within her when she gets pregnant. The annoying geek inside o' me could go on stating such facts forever, but you get the picture – your body is a fascinating piece of art.

Science has helped unravel most of the mysteries and captivating occurrences within your body – beginning from your general appearance and breaking it down to the tiniest molecules within you.

However, no matter how much we know, it's just not enough when it comes to the marvel that is the human body. Every day, we are at risk of facing the emergence of new mutant viral species and thus, science continues to evolve along with our problems and queries.

Could there be a cure for *AIDS*? Can we stop cancer? How can we develop a vaccine for *Hepatitis C*? All are genuine questions and are related to diseases or conditions that require a lot of attention today due to the toll they have taken on our lives and health.

Ageing can't be escaped so here's one question that hits us all: *Why do we tend to lose our memory as we age and can it be prevented?*

Is there a possibility that your loved ones (parents, grandparents, etc) could have been prevented from acquiring Alzheimer's disease[54]?

Can Schizophrenia be prevented by something in the diet?

Is there any simple and inexpensive way of boosting your problem-solving skills, memory and brain function?

Could your child's Autism be prevented or treated by something in his/her diet?

The good news is that science has found potentially strong answers to all the above questions in just one substance – Vitamin B12.[55]

The Background

Your nervous system is made up of the brain, the spinal cord and all the nerves in your body. The brain and the cord are the central nervous system whereas the nerves are the peripheral nervous system. Both are affected in different ways.

How B12 Deficiency Could Wreak Havoc in Your Nerves

Vitamin B12 is absolutely necessary for making the protective sheaths of all the neurones within your body. When these protective sheaths (called the **myelin** sheaths) are faulty or not made properly, your neurones will not be able to conduct nerve impulses properly. What does that mean?

Suppose you touch a hot object – your normal response would be to quickly draw back your hand. The nerves on the skin of your hand detect that you have touched something too hot which could damage your skin and therefore, they transmit this to your brain in the form of a nerve impulse. The brain 'orders' the muscles in your hand and arm to act in a way that results in your hand being drawn backwards – all this happens within a fraction of a second.

If these nerves weren't functioning well, imagine how hard it would be for you to feel simple things such as pain, pressure, heat, etc. In addition, when nerves get damaged, they start giving you funny feelings such as tingling sensations, pins and needles, etc. We all know how irritating it is when we sit in one position for too long and our arm or leg goes numb – only to give rise to that utterly annoying, indescribable feeling of 'pins and needles' in our skin. If you're not taking enough B12, you could find yourself in this vexing situation most of the time. Baaah.

How Low B12 Levels Could Shrink Your Brain[56]

Sounds crazy, I know. But that's the literal interpretation to what really happens to the brains of those who miss out on this super-vitamin. With low B12 levels, your brain substance decreases, making it very hard for the brain to conduct the nerve impulses to various parts of your body for giving it orders and directing it what to do.

The brain controls everything in your body so you could be thinking 'damn, does that mean any part of my brain could be affected and I could suffer from just about any type of symptom?' Genuine question, however, only certain parts are affected and going into the details of which ones are affected and why will put you to sleep (trust me, as much as I love neurology, studying those pathways and mugging up the anatomy really did put my patience to the test – I see the medical student agrees with me!)

All you need to know is that if you're not taking enough B12, your brain mass will decrease and you'll find yourself in a state of confusion most of the times. You won't be able to remember things or maintain a good attention span.

The reason behind that is twofold. Firstly, B12 helps form the protective coating on many parts of your nervous system, including the brain and nerves. Secondly, it is also involved in the metabolism of homocysteine, a very bad substance for both your heart and brain if not present within its normal limits. When you don't take B12, this substance will increase in your body, making you moody as well as directly causing your brain mass to decrease. [57]

Moody? Take Some B12[58]

I don't only hate feeling low, I even dislike the certain times when I feel manic. Oh no, I'm definitely not suffering from any disorder such as

Bipolar Disorder or the likes – but I feel low when I haven't had some 'me' time in a long while and I feel high whenever I have too much caffeine.

Inconsistent moods or mood swings can be a nuisance to those suffering from them and just about anyone who witnesses such incidents. If you feel that you're depressed, lonely, losing interest in the things you usually enjoy or getting increasingly irritable – you might not be taking enough B12.[59]

Again, our old friend homocysteine is the bad guy here[60]. High levels of this substance aren't going to do your psychological state any good[61] so get your hands on some B12[62] (AFTER consulting your doctor).

Ageing and Memory Issues? Take Some B12! [63]

As we age, homocysteine (yes, that same old bad guy I keep ranting about) starts to accumulate in our body due to multiple factors and leads to loss of brain matter which, in turn, causes memory loss as well as low cognition.[64]

Before it comes to get you, keep your forces prepared and stock up on B12 by consuming a healthy diet and/or taking regular supplements to stop and/or slow down the loss of your memory.

Tripping? Could Be a B12 Deficiency!

Been tripping a lot lately? Finding it hard to balance yourself and perform simple tasks like walking in the dark or washing your hair? In case you're not imagining things, it's time for you to consult your doctor and tell him/her about your symptoms in detail.

Such symptoms are a marker of an advanced B12 deficiency and will usually be accompanied by symptoms of anaemia, which I described earlier. If you don't get treated IMMEDIATELY for these symptoms, you could develop permanent paralysis which would be untreatable.

In addition, depending on the degree of damage to your nervous system, you could have other symptoms such as loss of vibration sense in your legs, problems coordinating and something known as hyperreflexia.

Hyperreflexia is a condition in which your muscular responses become exaggerated – something that your doctor will be able to demonstrate. When it comes to the nervous system, things can't always be predicted when it comes to the exact area which will be involved due to some disease or damage – therefore, you could have a multitude of varying symptoms, no two people usually having exactly the same symptoms.

The reason why I'm telling you this is that it's no use looking up your symptoms online trying to find a diagnosis by finding similarities with others who might have had such symptoms – you can get a general overview as to how they develop but your doctor is the ultimate source for the definitive diagnosis.

Is The World Spinning?! Might Be a B12 Deficiency

That's something called vertigo, where you feel that the world around you is actually spinning and you won't be able to balance yourself if you try to move a lot or stand up. Your eyes, ears and sensors in your body help your brain decide the right posture for you, making you see your surroundings the way they are in reality and adjusting your position accordingly.

The nerves in your ears that carry these 'sensations' to your brain can be damaged by a B12 deficiency, making you feel like everything's going round and round around you. In addition, you might get hearing problems – all of these turning into permanent issues if you don't get treated on time.

Bladder Problems? Could It Be a B12 Deficiency?

Although it's very highly unlikely for you to have ONLY bladder issues if you have a B12 deficiency, there are good chances for you to have such issues if you have the symptoms of anaemia and/or the other neurological symptoms I described above.

This, and a couple of other symptoms (listed after this) arise due to the malfunction of the autonomic nervous system – a part of the nervous system that basically controls mostly those functions of your body that you are not conscious about, such as digestion, heart activity, excretion, etc.

That makes it a pretty major system. There's a part of this system that helps you manage stress, meaning it speeds up your heart and diverts your blood to your brain and muscles when you need it, for example, in cases where you have to run from a lion (or in less dramatic circumstances, when you're taking an exam).

How does B12 deficiency cause problems with this system? The same old theory of the protective neuronal sheaths applies here too, so that the nerves of this part of the nervous system won't be functioning well and thus, you won't able to control your voiding habits. So hey, before it becomes too late, consult your doctor. If this situation stays for too long, you might have irreversible damage to your nervous system.

Droopy Eyelids or Double Vision?

The eyes are a unique organ – doctors can look directly into your eyes to judge the state of your brain (in many disease conditions). The eye is the only organ in the body which lets doctors see the state of your blood vessels (without cutting you open, as in surgeries).

What's even more fascinating is that the nerve of the eye – the optic nerve is a direct continuation of the brain. Anything that affects the eye can travel up the brain directly and vice versa. In addition, it's just a nerve – meaning low B12 levels could strip it off of its protective sheath.

That would mess up your vision and in fairly advanced stages, could lead to something called tunnel vision. In this condition, you will only see what's right in front of you, not what's on the sides, as if you were looking through a tunnel.

Moreover, the muscles of the eyes work through nerves, just like all other muscles of your body. If their nerves get messed up, they will act asynchronously or won't act at all – that could cause your eyelids to droop (and block your vision) or make you experience double vision (which could be a constant source of headache).

When you go to an eye specialist, he or she might or might not carry out B12 tests (since other diseases can easily mimic this disorder) so don't forget to remind your doctor. You should be certain that you had this easily treatable condition ruled out from the causes of your current symptoms.

For Geeks Only: What Causes Tunnel Vision?

How come people lose their peripheral vision? Why don't they lose their central vision first? That's because of the blood supply to the nerve fibres in the retina as well the arrangement of the fibres – those at the periphery are affected first and those in the centre are affected in later stages because of their better blood supply.

Can't Swallow Properly? Is B12 Deficiency the Cause?

Wherever there are nerves, there is a constant need of B12 to keep their protective sheaths intact so they can conduct nerve impulses. If they don't get what they want (B12 in this case), they won't be very nice to you.

They won't let you swallow properly – food could get stuck or you might have to put in some extra effort to gulp down whatever you eat. Pretty frustrating if you ask me. Trust me, it could get worse.

The body is fascinating as it is, but any tiny thing going missing or malfunctioning within it could affect just about any part of your body. Look what the deficiency of just a vitamin could end up doing to you! That makes it much more than 'just a vitamin'.

Symptoms Caused When B12 Deficiency Affects Your Nerves

Now that I feel that I have scared you enough when it comes to what B12 deficiency could do to your nervous system, let's have a look at all the symptoms that could arise due to problems with this particular organ system when B12 isn't enough in your body.

Depression
Anxiety
Irritability
Difficulty concentrating
Short-term memory loss
Moodiness
Low concentration span
Difficulty concentrating or getting familiar with new concepts
Difficulty walking and/or clumsiness
Tingling, numbness or 'pins and needles' sensations
Eye Problems (tunnel vision, droopy eyelids, double vision, etc)

Bladder problems
Difficulty swallowing
Difficulty balancing yourself

B12 Deficiency and Your Child: From Brain Injury to Autism
Adults have large stores of B12 in their liver and it generally takes about 7 years on average for signs of B12 deficiency to appear in them. However, children do not have the same amounts of stored B12 and therefore, their symptoms will appear sooner than they do in adults. [65]

The human body is prone to numerous disorders at both extremes of age – the details of which could fill up volumes of books – so let's just stick to your child's nervous system right now and see why it's so important to keep your child from being B12 deficient.

Your nervous system is not well-developed when you're born. Maximum development of the nervous system happens in the first few years of life and any problems in this time period leave a PERMANENT deficit in the child. An example is that of cortical blindness.

This is a condition in which the eye is perfectly normal but during the first few years of life, benign and easily treatable problems in the eye cause both the eyes to see a different image (for example, one eye could have problems seeing distant objects while the other eye is normal).
In such cases, the child's brain will process only one image and suppress the one from the faulty eye. If this continues for too long, the part in the brain that processes images will become permanently insensitive to images from that faulty eye. That will make the child blind in that eye forever, even though the eye is normal.

In other words, his brain would be blind to what his eye sees because all images are processed in the brain and that's where we finally perceive whatever we see. If an adult has a problem in one eye, he will notice it and get headaches due to the different images formed in both eyes. He won't go blind because his brain is already developed.

Similarly, if your child is not getting enough B12 in his diet, his nervous system will fail to develop properly.[66] If an adult is deprived of B12, his nervous system DETERIORATES, while a child's nervous system would

FAIL TO DEVELOP in similar circumstances.

He will fail to grow as other children of the same age group and will experience developmental delay – meaning your child won't walk or talk or sit up at the expected age.

In addition, he might get permanent brain damage that will cause muscular paralysis, learning deficits and even autism. The biochemical reason behind this is the same as that in the adult but the developmental state of your child is what makes it different.

Remember that your child will not be able to tell you what he/she feels – keep a close watch on his developmental milestones in consultation with his or her paediatrician. Infancy and childhood are times of high metabolism and since all organs are growing, a child's nutritional needs have to be kept in mind and satisfied accordingly because nutritional deficiencies can cause permanent problems in children (in addition to numerous other conditions, probably beyond the scope of your patience, not just this book!).

Here are the symptoms your child could have if his nervous system isn't getting the required amounts of B12:

Irritability
Problems walking
Numbness
Tingling
Confusion
Eyesight issues

(Symptoms of Anaemia will probably be present along with all these symptoms and include pale skin, cracks at the angles of the mouth, sore tongue, increased heart rate, fatigue, difficulty feeding, etc).

Ageing and B12 Deficiency
Could these set the stage for the development of Alzheimer's disease?

So now you know for sure that B12 is strongly related to the health of your nervous system. I only discussed your peripheral nerves in the story above – but that's not all. B12 deficiency directly affects your brain, as explained earlier. However, this statement does not explain much. That's because it doesn't tell you that as you age, you are more likely to develop a B12 deficiency even if you're getting enough in your diet, and this deficiency might set the stage for the development of Alzheimer's disease.

The question is why?

The elderly are at a greater risk of malabsorption of B12 from their diets (principally because conditions such as atrophic gastritis, etc affect this group more than other age groups). That increases the levels of homocysteine in your blood – a substance that causes decline of mental function along with raising the risk of heart attacks and altering your mood.

A few years ago, the *National Institute of Ageing* funded a study conducted by *Dr. Christine C. Tangney* in which 121 people from Chicago who were 65 years or older were included. B12 tests as well as mental functions were assessed in the beginning. Approximately 4.5 years later, MRI scans of their brains were carried out in addition to testing the markers of B12 deficiency.

It was found that those who had 4 or 5 markers of B12 deficiency had lower scores on mental function tests (such as cognitive skills, memory, etc). The MRI scans showed that those who were deficient also had lower brain volume as compared to their normal counterparts.

The average score on the cognitive function tests was 0.23 and the range was -2.18 to +1.42. Interestingly, it was noted that with increasing levels of homocysteine in the blood, cognitive functions declined (every one micromole per litre of homocysteine caused a decline in the mental function test scores by 0.03 marks).

Dr. Christine C. Tangney said that it wasn't the deficiency of B12 itself but a rise in its markers, such as homocysteine that caused the mentioned effects on the brain. She also said:

"Our findings definitely deserve further examination. It's too early to say whether increasing vitamin B12 levels in older people through diet or

50

supplements could prevent these problems, but it is an interesting question to explore. Findings from a British trial with B vitamin supplementation are also supportive of these outcomes."

So although more research is needed to prove how this association is caused and whether it needs to be dealt with on a wide-scale level, you now know that B12 deficiency definitely DOES put you at risk for developing memory loss, low mental function and eventually even Alzheimer's disease as you age.

If your B12 levels are low before you approach old age, you might even get Alzheimer's or memory loss before the expected age – something called 'early onset Alzheimer's disease.'

It is not certain that your body will have both the symptoms of anaemia and impaired neurological function so don't ignore your symptoms thinking that they are not severe enough or should be accompanied by those of anaemia. You can have all the neurological symptoms listed earlier.

If your mental function is declining, you will experience:

1. Short term memory loss (meaning you will remember what happened in your childhood but won't be able to recall whether you brushed your hair 5 minutes ago or not).
2. Failure to concentrate.
3. Problems grasping new concepts or taking too long to learn anything new.
4. Problems coordinating.
5. Walking problems and failure to balance yourself.
6. Problems while communicating (mainly because you won't remember what you said a few moments ago).
7. Hallucinations/imagining things.
8. Emotional instability or moodiness.
9. A tendency to misplace things.

Vitamin B12 Deficiency and Heart Disease

Low levels of B12 cause high levels of homocysteine – the substance that is the reason behind the association between B12 deficiency and heart disease (along with deficiencies of Vitamins B6 and B9)

Homocysteine Homocysteine Homocysteine! Of course by now you're wondering if it's just you or if I actually might have an obsession with this substance. Hey, don't blame me guys, it just keeps coming in my way when I'm looking into how B12 deficiency is involved in causing brain shrinkage and heart problems.

So before we get into further details regarding your heart, let's get to know homocysteine a little better and then see why it causes heart disease.

What is Homocysteine ?

Homocysteine is an amino acid – a building block for the proteins in your body (meaning your muscles, the membranes of your cells, antibodies, etc). It is made from another amino acid, methionine.

What Causes High Homocysteine Levels?

Low amounts of Vitamins B6, B9 and B12 are all associated with this condition[67].Moreover, diets high in proteins, such as meats (since these contain high amounts of methionine) are also correlated with increased levels of homocysteine in addition to some genetic conditions which result n faulty metabolism of homocysteine and thus, raised levels in the blood. In addition, obesity, smoking, alcohol, a sedentary lifestyle and certain drugs (such as the diabetes drug *metformin*, etc) are also contributory factors.

How Does Homocysteine Cause Heart Disease?[68]

Oxidative stress and inflammation[69] are modernity's possible worst enemy - and a high level of homocysteine is perhaps one of the strongest markers for chronic inflammation and oxidative stress. By damaging the lining of your blood vessels, homocysteine causes thickening of your arteries by promoting atherosclerosis[70] as well as blood clots since damage to the arteries is an inciting factor for both these events. [71]

With both these problems[72], the risk of coronary heart disease (where the blood vessels that supply the heart get narrowed and thus the heart's nutrition is compromised and parts of its muscle can die, causing a heart attack as well as chronic heart disease) greatly rises.

Can Heart Disease Be Prevented By Lowering Homocysteine Levels?

A number of studies have been conducted to find out whether low homocysteine levels could prevent heart disease but the American Heart Association still hasn't confirmed whether low homocysteine levels could really prevent heart disease.

Some studies contradict this[73] whereas some are in its favour. [74]That means there's some more research required to find out about this association. On the other hand, we do know for sure that high homocysteine levels cause heart disease.

What Can You Do to Lower Your Homocysteine Levels?

Follow a healthy diet composed mainly of vegetables and grass-fed clean animal products. You'll get plenty of B-vitamins[75] along with the rest of the required nutrition. Make sure you work out (high-intensity workouts are preferred) and avoid smoking and excessive alcohol intake. Consult your doctor to begin supplements if you have any of the predisposing factors for elevated homocysteine levels (see below).

Who Is at Risk for Developing High Homocysteine Levels?

People who do not have enough of the B vitamins in their diet

Elderly individuals (because they have a higher chance of suffering from malabsorption of the B-vitamins).

People who are taking drugs such as metformin (for Diabetes), Levodopa (for Parkinson's disease), Phenytoin (for Epilepsy) etc.

People who consume too much caffeine (present in chocolates, fizzy drinks, energy drinks and coffee).

People who consume alcohol and/or smoke.

People who do not have a healthy lifestyle and do not exercise regularly.

People who have chronic renal disease (mainly because the kidneys won't be able to flush out homocysteine and it will build up in the blood).

Does Homocysteine Cause Other Diseases?

In addition to heart disease, you might recall that homocysteine causes Alzheimer's disease and brain shrinkage (brain atrophy).

It has also been linked[76] numerous times[77] again and again[78] with the development of **migraine**[79] and **stroke,** the latter association being due to the effect on the blood vessels. When vessels become narrow due to atherosclerosis, they are prone to getting blocked by clots or not being able to supply nutrients and oxygen to your brain – something that causes brain dysfunction and death of brain tissue. That is cerebrovascular accident (CVA) or stroke.

High levels of homocysteine have also been associated with a greater risk of developing macular degeneration – a condition of the eyes where the retina (or the layer within the eye that processes and transmits images to the brain) begins to degenerate[80].One study even found out that this disabling condition can be prevented by therapy with Vitamin B12, amongst other nutrients.[81]

To sum up, you need to remember that the B vitamins lower the levels of homocysteine, preventing numerous disorders. So do not miss out on any of them.

When it comes to homocysteine, research is still being carried out and we need more evidence to find out particular facts as to how much of the vitamins are required to effectively prevent all the mentioned diseases – until then, let's make sure we are getting enough of these vitamins in our diets since research can take decades and life's too short to keep waiting! Utilise the evidence that we do have and stick to a healthy diet plan.

B12 Deficiency and Your Immune System

If you remember B12's functions, understanding this bit will be very easy for you. Remember that B12 is involved in DNA formation as well as the maintenance and stability of your cell membranes? Another thing I mentioned in its functions was how it helps bind certain molecules on the membranes of your cells – these molecules act as markers that tell your immune system not to attack them. That's why it attacks only foreign cells or substances, not your own cells.

If you're deficient in B12, you could develop problems with your immune system.[82] These problems can be of three types:

Increased Infections:

Because B12 is needed for producing DNA and because actively dividing cells need more of it, tissues such as bone marrow and the lining of your gastrointestinal tract will be affected early (since the cells of these tissues divide much more than other cells in your body).

Your bone marrow makes all the cells present in your blood, including the white blood cells or the cells of the immune system which fight infections. Our daily activities bring numerous germs into contact with us but we don't get active infection because the white blood cells produced by our bone marrow kill these germs by launching an active immune response against them.

When you don't take enough B12, your marrow won't be able to make the lots of DNA that it needs for the production of white blood cells. Therefore, the white blood cells produced will be immature (a similar situation to that encountered by the red blood cells, if you recall).

These immature white blood cells have a shorter life span as compared to their normal counterparts – thus putting you at risk of developing infections due to the low counts of immature white blood cells.

Autoimmune Disorders:

These are conditions in which a person's immune system fails to recognise the cells of his or her own body, attacking them 'thinking' they are foreign. Various organs are attacked in different types of diseases, the details of which are not necessary here.

What you need to know is that B12 deficiency causes malfunctioning of the cell membranes of your cells, which can lead to loss of the markers on your cells which ward off white blood cells telling them that they belong to your body and should not be attacked.

With loss of B12, these markers are lost and your cells are liable to attack by your immune system. Trust me, it's not a pretty state when your own army launches an attack on you – just about any organ can be attacked and the results can even be fatal sometimes.

Another thing you need to know is that B12 deficiency and autoimmune conditions go hand-in-hand – an autoimmune disorder such as pernicious anaemia causes B12 deficiency itself whereas a pre-existing autoimmune disorder, such as *Hashimoto's thyroiditis* (a condition of your thyroid gland) can put a person at risk for the development of a vitamin B12 deficiency.

Interestingly, low thyroid function might itself be caused a B12 deficiency. All you need to remember is that it works both ways because B12 maintains healthy cell membranes – the structures that contain the receptors for many of your hormones. No B12 means faulty cell membranes that won't be able to hold those receptors, therefore no hormones will get into your cells to cause the actions they were meant to produce. What a shame for all those chemicals to go to waste. It's a cruel world we live in.

Let's look at the conditions associated with B12 deficiency:

Pernicious Anaemia:[83] Described earlier multiple times, this condition causes your immune system to attack the cells of your stomach that produce intrinsic factor, the substance required for the absorption of vitamin B12.

Autoimmune Thyroiditis: [84]This is a condition that can affect your thyroid gland and causes low levels of thyroid hormone, a chemical responsible for metabolism, energy production, growth and development, etc.

People who have this condition are at high risk of developing B12 deficiency due to Pernicious Anaemia. If you have this condition, your thyroid will gradually get destroyed and you will experience the symptoms of *hypothyroidism* (discussed in more details in the section on endocrine problems associated with B12 deficiency).

Addison's disease:[85] This occurs when the adrenal glands (triangular glands sitting on top of each of your kidneys, responsible for secreting hormones that influence and/or control your blood pressure, heart rate, sexual characteristics as well sexual functions and help your body deal with stress and infections) get destroyed or start to malfunction.

People who have this condition are also at high risk of developing pernicious anaemia. Addison's disease causes lethargy, weakness, abdominal pain, vomiting, diarrhoea, depression, etc.

All the symptoms are due to low or absent production of cortisol (a steroid that increases blood sugar levels and helps you counter stress, apart from making you feel happy and cheerful) and aldosterone (a hormone that monitors how much water you lose in your urine, increasing the absorption of water into the body and helping to increase blood pressure when it's below normal limits).

Poor Response to Vaccines:

When you're given vaccines, your body makes antibodies to these and 'remembers' the germ that was part of the vaccine, forming the same antibodies to it when you get that germ in your body the next time, due to an infection.

B12 deficiency causes an improper formation of antibodies due to which the vaccines you get won't work properly. You'll be thinking that you've got your vaccine shots and are immune but you'll fall ill when you're exposed to that particular germ!

Chronic Diarrhoea or Indigestion? Vitamin B12 & Your Gastrointestinal Tract

You probably remember how I went on and on about how B12 deficiency affects the fastest growing cells first. That's why your gastrointestinal system can be affected causing vague symptoms such as:

Diarrhoea

Indigestion

Bloating

Abdominal discomfort

Abdominal Pain

If you've been having such symptoms for quite some time and your doctor hasn't been able to figure out what's wrong with you, you definitely need to tell him/her to consider testing you for B12 deficiency.

Vitamin B12 and Your Musculoskeletal System
Although it's not known how or why low B12 causes it, studies have

found that this deficiency is a possible risk factor for the development of osteoporosis. That's a condition due to which bone density decreases but the composition of the bone remains unaffected. That will cause bone pains, weak bones which fracture easily, etc. In addition, low B12 deficiency will also cause muscular pains and cramps

Vitamin B12 Deficiency and Your Skin

Since B12 is required for rapidly growing cells (which includes those of the skin), this organ of your body can be affected by B12 deficiency with vague symptoms such as rashes, itching, hair loss and tingling. Time to get a B12 test if you have these problems.

Bruising an Bleeding Problems

Your bone marrow produces cells called platelets which are involved in forming clots and healing wounds. With low B12 levels, marrow function is compromised as explained earlier and therefore, platelets decrease in number – a condition called *thrombocytopenia*.

The symptoms of this problem are:

Easy bruising

Small, red marks on your skin (which indicate bleeding sites in or under your skin which take too long to heal)

Delayed healing of wounds

Excessive bleeding from cuts which takes too long to stop

Bleeding from the gums when your brush your teeth

If not treated on time, anyone who has low platelets can start bleeding within their own body and very urgent and intensive treatment would be required to save their life.

Reproductive Problems in Men

Low levels have been associated with impaired fertility in men – that's because adequate amounts of B12 are required to sustain development of growing cells. Sperms are constantly replenished and need good motility to travel up in the uterus to be able to fertilise the ovum. However, further evidence needs to be collected regarding this theory and other possible mechanisms.

There have been only a few studies on this subject and therefore, a definite association is still to be found. However, if you're having problems when it comes to the fertility department, you should definitely have a good and healthy diet – it is the basic pre-requisite for the production of healthy sperms.

It is strongly speculated that vitamin B12 raises sperm count – how or why this happens is still to be found. Before you begin any supplements, do not forget to consult your doctor about this.

Reproductive Problems in Women

Feeling blue or experiencing problems during your menstrual cycle? Maybe it's a B12 deficiency!

Many women are affected by PMS or premenstrual syndrome – a handful of annoying symptoms like lethargy, depression, insomnia or excessive somnolence, etc. This happens around 5-11 days before the beginning of each menstrual cycle. Yes, that means every single month and for those of the women affected by it, a major part of their lives is taken up dealing with this issue. If you're one of them, of course you want to get rid of it. Doctors give hormonal contraceptives or antidepressants to help control your symptoms but this can result in recurrence of your symptoms.

Another much worse, closely related condition is PMDD (*premenstrual dysphoric disorder*) in which all the symptoms of premenstrual syndrome are heightened in intensity. It can be very hard to cope with and patients might even have to be put on anti-depressants.

If this were a one-time problem, of course women would just sleep through it and forget it ever happened. But sadly, people with this condition have to deal with it for half their lives (till they reach their menopause) – so naturally any measure that helps reduce these symptoms is welcome.

Well for those of you who do have these issues, B12 might be the good news that you've been waiting for.

There's a lot of theories as to how low B12 levels could cause these symptoms, some of which include: B12 affects your hormones (as explained in the section on the endocrine system) along with metabolising homocysteine (the chemical that causes low moods) and being involved in synthesising the neurotransmitters that control your mood (such as dopamine, serotonin, etc).

The association definitely exists but we cannot say for sure how or why B12 can help those with PMS and even PMDD. Consult your doctor before you start supplements – high doses will generally be required to be taken for a couple of months before signs of improvement appear.

In addition, those women who have irregular menstrual cycles (they bleed too much, too little, too early or too late) can also benefit from B12 supplementation. Wundabar!.. you've just exclaimed with great relish - a wonder vitamin indeed.

Problems Conceiving? B12 Might Be The Answer

Numerous couples go through terrible ordeals, spending thousands of dollars on expensive treatments, trying out exercises and new diet plans, visiting various infertility specialists – only to be disappointed again and again. Some of them do conceive but experience miscarriages or spontaneous abortions.

If you're one of them and you have not been diagnosed with any particular problem that could be causing this problem – it's time for another consultation to discuss B12 shots.[86]

Again, why and how B12 promotes and ensures a healthy conception is not fully understood but the association has been proven by research.[87] Of course, this is not the cure to your undiagnosed condition – all I'm trying to do is alert you to another possibility that is vitamin B12 deficiency, a condition readily and easily treatable.

The irony in that is the fact that this condition remains widely undiagnosed and untreated all because medical authorities haven't revised the respective outlines and guidelines that would bring the urgently needed 'revolution' in this regard. Until that happens, let's help ourselves while we can and seek the great aid of B12 shots.

B12 Deficiency and the Endocrine System

OF COURSE you know that B12 is needed to maintain healthy membranes and OF COURSE you also know that cell membranes have the receptors that internalise hormones from your blood into your cells. I've bugged you enough about that so let's just get to the main issue here.

B12 deficiency can cause hormonal problems by affecting just about any gland in your body. Here are the symptoms you can experience if you've got any of the mentioned conditions of hormonal imbalance:

Hypothyroidism ('Hypo' means low, so this word means low or decreased function of the thyroid gland):

Hair fall, Weight gain, Lethargy, Excessive somnolence, Dry and scaly skin, Low heart rate, Constipation, Depression, Low concentration span, Cold intolerance.

Since the thyroid gland (located in the front of your lung pipe or trachea, in your neck) is responsible for energy production, metabolism, growth and development, etc, a decrease in its function obviously leads to reversal of all those normal functions.

Both B12 deficiency and low thyroid function are closely related, each of them directly influencing the other. Therefore, either of them could cause the other one to appear in your body. Those who have thyroid diseases such as *Hashimoto's* or *Grave's* are at a very high risk of developing a B12 deficiency.

Hashimoto's thyroiditis will present with the symptoms described above, whereas Grave's disease produces symptoms opposite to those, i.e, increased heart rate, insomnia, weight loss, etc – all due to increased metabolic rate and an over-activity of the cells that respond to thyroid hormone.

Diabetes Mellitus

61

Diabetes can lead to B12 deficiency. In **type I diabetes**, the cells of the pancreas that produce insulin (the chemical that controls your blood sugar levels) are destroyed and thus, the affected patients are dependent on insulin administration for the rest of their lives.

In **type II Diabetes**, these cells are initially normal but the body develops resistance to Insulin and the body's cells don't take it up (Insulin helps the cells in your body to take in glucose and use it for energy production) even though glucose as well as insulin will be present in the blood.

Treatment of this disorder is aimed at reducing blood glucose levels as well lowering the body's resistance towards insulin. The drug *Metformin* causes B12 deficiency and on the other hand, auto-immune Diabetes or type I Diabetes is sometimes associated with Pernicious Anaemia which is a direct cause of B12 Deficiency.

Numerous other disorders such as Vitilogo, Crohn's disease, Ulcerative colitis, etc are associated with B12 deficiency – as explained in the causes of this condition in Chapter 2.

Could B12 Prevent Cancer?
Theoretically, hell yes! [88]

You already know that vitamin B12 is involved in making the DNA in your cells. Cancer cells have faulty DNA – the genes that go 'wrong' are what make the cells divide and behave in an abnormal fashion, not letting them do the work they were destined to carry out.

They turn into uncontrollable cells that divide on their will and seem to be autonomous. So when does B12 come in? According to a study, vitamin B12 causes these abnormal cells to commit suicide by letting them know they are not normal.

Exactly how it does so and what levels are required to achieve such miraculous results is a question I can't wait to have an answer to. The research associated with these facts was carried on mice, which is why I said that it is theoretically possible for B12 to 'cure' and/or prevent cancer. Although more research is definitely required in this field, it is definitely a promising one! I've totally got my fingers crossed

Unimaginable Consequences

If you've been having doubts about getting your B12 levels checked and you actually are suffering from it, things could get much worse for you in certain situations. In these special circumstances, the pre-existing B12 deficiency could lead to irreversible damage. Think I'm being melodramatic? Check out the section below and allow me to change your mind:

B12 Deficiency and Surgery

'Yeah, so what if I have a mild depression sometimes along with indigestion, lethargy and problems concentrating – it's probably the fact that I've crossed middle age.'

In case you're telling yourself things such as these to procrastinate tests of your B12 levels, you're going to end up with irreversible damage to your nervous system if you have to go through a surgery.[89]

Now, why would that be? That's because *Nitrous Oxide*, a substance used both in surgeries to anaesthetise patients and in street racing, combined with B12 and renders it ineffective. In people with normal B12 levels, this doesn't cause problems. In those with undiagnosed or even mild B12 deficiency, the dangerously low levels of B12 will be lost owing to the reaction with Nitrous Oxide, causing damage to the nervous system.

Symptoms of that are the same as those described in the section on how B12 deficiency effects your nervous system. However, these symptoms can appear within days to weeks of the surgery and are usually very hard to treat (large doses of B12 are required to do so) and the recovery is extremely slow, even incomplete in some cases.

So if you're sitting around, delaying your B12 tests even if you have a reason (I don't think any reason would be sound enough to make you delay these crucial tests), be sure to get this test before you get any surgery because doctors just might not remember.

B12 Deficiency and Pregnancy

When you're pregnant, you need to take in calories and nutrients for yourself as well the other tiny human inside you. If you don't take enough for the both of you, some nutrients will be drawn out from your stores so that the baby has enough of them. In time, you will run out of these nutrients if you do not replenish your stores. If you are already deficient in vitamin B12, you won't have adequate stores and the foetus won't get the amount of B12 that it (he?) requires for the development of its organ systems.[90]

When that happens, multiple birth defects could result in your baby because B12 is required for the synthesis of DNA – something that you baby needs in all of the cells that are continuing to grow and evolve in this baby. Your baby could develop neural tube defects, similar to what happens in folic acid deficiency. Due to this defect, the vertebral column does not form properly and there are problems in the spinal cord or even the brain itself, causing neurological issues in the baby.

It all depends on the extent of the malformation, some children might have an open vertebral canal with no neurological problem whereas others might have problems in the nerves supplying the limbs, thus taking away their ability to walk or move their legs.

Yes, that means that if you don't fix your B12 or folate deficiency before getting pregnant or don't take enough of these during the pregnancy, you could end up taking away your child's ability to walk (in addition to other possible defects such as bladder problems and in severe cases, absence of the brain itself, something that is not compatible with life).

Therefore, before you decide to get pregnant, get your B12 levels checked and get your deficiency treated as soon as possible to save yourself from the disappointment of having caused such disastrous consequences to your baby's health[91] – all due to failure to take in the required nutrients.

Remember to take in an absolute minimum 2.6 mcg of B12 during pregnancy every day. If you're deficient, you will need higher doses, so consult your doctor if you think you might have any symptoms of B12 deficiency.

B12 Deficiency When Breastfeeding

Babies up to the age of 4-6 months rely solely on milk. Those babies who are fed only by their mothers only have their mothers' milk for getting all the nutrients they need which is how they get the required amount of B12.

If a breastfeeding mother gets deficient in B12, she will not have notable symptoms in the early stages but her baby will begin to develop B12 deficiency. As I explained earlier in this chapter, babies don't have stores of B12 like adults do and they are much more susceptible to getting deficient as well as developing neurological symptoms if they do not get enough B12. [92]

Your infant's symptoms could be mild and you might not even notice them, but these set the stage for IRREVERSIBLE brain and nerve damage, leaving your child physically and mentally impaired for life.[93] Do you want to do that to you child? Obviously not. So if you're a vegetarian mother and you're breastfeeding your baby, don't forget to take enough supplements so that your child does not suffer the consequences of this easily preventable disorder.[94] Healthy women need 2.8 mcg of B12 daily whereas those who are deficient will need higher doses.

Does B12 Really Give You Energy?

Celebrities like Madonna, Katy Perry, Justin Timberlake and Victoria Beckam use B12 shots on the basis that it helps boost their energy. Even Margaret Thatcher used it for the same reasons. Does it really give them energy?

According to them, yes. However, there is no scientific evidence behind this fact. The simple explanation is that B12 is involved in the production of energy in your body – when you don't have enough B12, you won't get that energy and you'll feel lethargic. When you have enough of this vitamin, your energy levels will be just normal, not above that. Therefore, if you're not deficient in B12, you won't experience an energy boost. [51]

Consider the example of any machine that runs on some sort of fuel. Without fuel, it won't work but giving it extra fuel won't make it work better. Similarly, taking B12 only maintains our energy stores, it does not boost them. It only does so in cases of a deficiency.

Does B12 Help in Weight Loss?
Again, another use of B12 that you will come across in advertisements is, drums please – weight loss. Some parties claim that B12 aids in weight loss. However, this not totally true. You see, a higher-metabolism burns out more energy, and that might help you lose more weight, yes. But as we said just a paragraph ago, it can't 'over-energize' you more if you're not deficient.

B12 helps your body utilize the energy it has stored – it does not help you over-utilise those stores so that you might lose weight. Until such claims are supported by solid evidence, we cannot begin supplementation for the mere purpose of weight loss.

Those who claim that this vitamin has helped them reduce weight might be practising other methods of weight loss (without really knowing it), which is why proper research has to be undertaken to investigate on this particular fact. Until then, hit the gym please.

Chapter 4: The Diagnosis of Vitamin B12 Deficiency

For Doctors and Patients

Whether you're a doctor or just someone concerned about your health, you should know that...

With the current dismal state of affairs regarding the diagnosis of B12 deficiency, this chapter should be of utmost important to both the physician as well as the layman. It works both ways since this particular condition isn't thoroughly known amongst the general practitioners.

If you go to your doctor without any clue about what you might have and he/she does not include B12 deficiency in the differential diagnosis, you would suffer a lot if you actually do have this condition. You'd get one test after another, not to mention the physical and mental ordeal you will be put through.

However, being a doctor myself, it's sometimes very frustrating when our patients think they know more than us and keep insisting on getting some form of treatment when it might actually harm them or be of no use at all.

Therefore, do not argue with your doctors unnecessarily without really knowing what you're talking about. Base your queries on actual scientific evidence. If you read something online, ask your doctor about it.

Next, for the doctors – do not ignore what your patients ask you. The internet has made all sorts of information, whether it is right or wrong, easily accessible to the layman. Without a background in medical education, he may not be able to understand it all and could end up perceiving it in a rather distorted fashion.

Explain in detail and reinforce your answers with diagrams, flow charts or reliable sources that you can show the patients (such as research papers, etc). If you fail to do so, your patient might be unsatisfied with you, even if you've put him on the right treatment. Of course such things can be time consuming, but hey, such activities can keep your patient from trying out new things that he/she has read about on the internet, things we all know can have devastating consequences.

How Is a B12 Deficiency Usually Diagnosed

Physicians end up missing mild signs and symptoms of this condition. When they do suspect B12 deficiency, they go for serum B12 levels, homocysteine levels, etc.[95]

However, it's sad that many of them choose to ignore their patients' symptoms by relying solely on the laboratory tests. This is completely absurd since B12 deficiency is very easy to treat,[96] is inexpensive and B12 is nontoxic even in high amounts. So all you doctors out there, what's the big deal[97] in administering B12 to someone who MIGHT have its deficiency?

How _Should_ B12 Deficiency be Diagnosed?

(For those concerned with the medical profession)

For all those that have ended up in the medical profession, we need to open up some old-forgotten textbooks again and skim through the latest research to put an end to the notorious B12 deficiency by trying to diagnose it at its earliest. If you're not a physician, you will probably find it hard to go through this section.

You can skip it if you like, but remember what symptoms this deficiency can cause and what you need to be beware of. Another thing to remember is that you should always tell your physician all your symptoms; it is for your doctor to decide which symptoms are important and which ones aren't. Don't keep any signs and symptoms from your physicians thinking they're not as important as your 'main' symptom.

So, back to our question: How should B12 deficiency be diagnosed?

We clearly need to redefine this particular area of medicine since faults within physicians and/or the 'system' are the actual reason why B12 deficiency is under-diagnosed. This condition is much more prevalent than once believed.[98]

I strongly believe that a detailed history and examination make up about 70-80% of the diagnosis, or help you narrow your differential diagnosis to a few conditions which you can further confirm or rule out by the help of investigations. Therefore, you should take a detailed history, examine the patient thoroughly and THEN send them to get the required tests done.

When you get the test results back and they don't confirm the diagnosis of a B12 deficiency, don't think you can ignore your patients' symptoms because if left untreated, these symptoms could turn worse and might reflect irreversible damage. Keeping that in mind, here's how the suspicion of a B12 Deficiency should be approached (recall all the signs and symptoms of various organ systems as explained in chapters 2 and 3 respectively):

(Note: The following proposed protocol is based on the one provided by *Dr. Joseph Chandy*, GP for 44 years who has been working on B12 from the past 30 years, and his assistant, *Dr. Hugo Minney*, Ph. D on their B12 deficiency support group and charity at www.b12d.org. This protocol is highly extensive and is based on Dr. Chandy's experience with numerous patients of B12 deficiency over the past 3 decades.

Step 1 - Which presenting complaints or symptoms should alert you to a possible B12 Deficiency?

- Lethargy
-
- Tiredness

- Depression

- Hair loss

- Altered sensations in the limbs or pins and needles, numbness,etc

- Tremors and nerve palsies (such as facial palsy, oculomotor nerve palsy, etc).

- Dizziness, fainting spells and headaches which are frequent or recurrent

- Palpitations

Step 2 - If most or some of the above are bothering the patient, ask about the following in detail:

- Ask your patient about their diet – are they vegans?

- History of any similar in the family (to rule out prevalence of pernicious anaemia in their family)

- History of gastric surgery,

- History of ileal surgery,

- History of the usage of drugs that hamper B12 absorption (such as metformin, proton pump inhibitors, salicylates, etc)

- History of alcohol consumption (ask about how much alcohol the patient takes, when he takes it, for how long he has been doing so, etc).

Step 3: Ask your patient to grade his/her symptoms in the questionnaire (you can download here, print it and give to your patients whenever it's needed).

Here are a few things you need to know about the grading and how it will help you reach your diagnosis:

- Ask your patient to grade his/her symptoms out of a total score of 10

- A grade of 1 indicates that the patient has the particular symptom but is not bothered too much by it since that very symptom occurs very infrequently. A score of 5 indicates that the symptom is present on and off and bothers the patients only moderately. A score of 10 means that that particular symptom is present most or all of the time and is a constant source of annoyance or distress for the patient.

- When your patient is done, take the questionnaire and add up the scores of each system in the yellow bars.

- After you have done that, count the number of yellow bars (or involved systems) that have a score of 5 and above – the greater the number of systems involved, the more severe the deficiency of

B12.

Step 4 - Rule out other possible diseases:

Once the form gives you a clear idea of the involved systems, confirm the diagnosis of a vitamin B12 deficiency (before grading its severity) by performing a thorough examination and the appropriate investigations to exclude disorders that can mimic the symptoms your patient has.

Common tests include a complete blood profile, a blood smear, tests for folate deficiency, *multiple sclerosis, thyroiditis, Addison's* disease, *Alzheimer's* disease, *Coeliac* disease, specific tests for vitamin B12 deficiency and *Pernicious Anaemia* (explained in detail in the next section) etc.

Rule out all possible conditions before landing on the final diagnosis of B12 deficiency because although low B12 levels are easily treatable, the disorders that mimic B12 deficiency are not and if left untreated, severe morbidity or even mortality could result. Therefore, don't get enthusiastic about diagnosing B12 without looking into other possible causes, which when not found, should prompt you to begin B12 therapy.

Step 5 – Grade the severity of the B12 deficiency: In order to grade the severity of a B12 deficiency in your patient, use the chart from b12d.com along with the questionnaire your patient filled out and the result of his/her B12 tests.

Step 6 - Begin vitamin B12 therapy:

Based on what category your patient fits into, begin one of the following treatment regimens (taken from the protocol for excluding B12 deficiency by *Dr. Joseph Chandy and Dr. Hugo Minney*, on www.b12d.org):

B12 deficiency (Pernicious Anaemia) and other macrocytic anaemias without neurological involvement*.
Hydroxocobalamin or methylcobalamin Initially 1mg 3 times a week for 2 weeks then 1mg every 2-3 months.

B12 deficiency (Pernicious Anaemia) with neurological signs and symptoms*. Initially 1mg on alternate days until no further improvement (maximum reversal of neuro-psychiatric signs and symptoms are achieved), then 1mg every 1-2 months.

Prophylaxis or Therapeutic Trial. 1mg IM or SC (hydroxocobalamin or methylcobalamin) should be given   alternate days for 2 – 3 weeks (6 to 9 doses) followed by 1mg IM or SC5 per week for 3 months. If there is no improvement in signs and symptoms after 3 months (13 weeks) then B12 deficiency can be excluded. A   therapeutic trial will not interact with other medication given and other treatment can be started at the same time. Review treatment pathway after 3 months.

* Clinically review every 1 or 2 months with or without serum B12 and if clinically indicated, increase the frequency to every 2 *months, every month or more frequently.*

Tests Available for Detecting Vitamin B12 Deficiency

Tests Available for Detecting Vitamin B12 Deficiency

Numerous tests are available to confirm whether a person is suffering from a B12 deficiency or not. Let's look at them and see if healthcare professionals need to do something in order to change the way these tests are interpreted:

Serum B12 Levels:
As its name implies, this test is done to check the amount of B12 in your serum. As I mentioned earlier in Chapter 2, this range varies roughly from 200-900 pg/ml[99]. However, some hospitals have redefined these ranges into the following[100] –

Deficient <200pg/ml
Borderline 200-270pg/ml
Normal 271-870pg/ml

This method seems better because it considers those patients in the 'borderline' category and can serve well to diagnose and treat such patients before their symptoms worsen. However, these ranges still need to be revised.

In their book '*Could it be B12?*' Pacholok and *Stuart* write:

"We believe[101] that the "normal" serum B12 threshold needs to be raised from 200 pg/ml to at least **450 pg/ml** *because deficiencies begin to appear in the cerebrospinal fluid [102](CSF) below 550 pg/ml.[103]*

At this time, we believe normal serum B12 levels should be greater than 550 pg/ml. For brain and nervous system health and prevention of disease in older adults, serum B12 levels should be maintained near or above **1000 pg/ml.**

We commonly see patients with clinical signs of B12 deficiency who are not being tested. Others who are being tested are not being treated because their serum B12 falls in the grey zone. This error results in delayed diagnosis and an increased incidence of injury."

What does it all mean?
Let's divide that answer into two parts: One for the layman – the concerned mother, the worried grandson, the zealous fitness geek or just someone who's reading this thinking 'what's all the B12 hype about?'

The other one is for those in the medical profession.

For the layman:
All this information means that the values that have been seen in the labs for judging whether a person is B12 deficient or not, are misleading and are one of the major reasons why people are not being diagnosed with B12 deficiency when they most definitely might be suffering from it.

Therefore, urge your doctors to explain their reasons for not beginning a B12 deficiency treatment when you feel that you have its symptoms. You know now that their 'standards' for diagnosing B12 deficiency are not exactly correct, might as well do something about it!

Your physicians aren't exactly to be blamed for it; it's the 'system' and the way they're taught. It would take quite some time to bring changes in these particular areas but don't just wait around hoping for a revolution to come and magically end up diagnosing you and your loved ones.

You must make use of the information you have to save yourself from the crippling and oft irreversible damage done by this ridiculously easily treatable disorder.

For those in the medical profession:
Try to follow these ranges, instead of the standard ones you have been taught or the ones that your local labs follow:

Normal >550pg/ml

Deficient < 550pg/ml

Adequate to maintain a healthy nervous system and to prevent disease in elderly individuals 1000pg/ml
As you can clearly see, these particular ranges rule out those in the 'gray zone,' many of which according to   *Pacholok* and *Stuart*, end up without B12 therapy because their physicians don't consider them B12   deficient.

Think I'm over-doing it a bit? In that case, what about those countries whose normal serum B12 levels are defined to be at least at 500 pg/ml? These countries include Japan and a few European countries – so if some of us have already accepted the proposed revisions of normal B12 levels, why can't we all?

Until your countries carry out such efforts, don't ignore your patients based on mere 'lab standards.' Medical standards are set to diagnose and treat patients – if they're not helping you do that, the purpose is lost and it's time for you to redefine those standards. In addition, B12 serum levels shouldn't be the ONLY thing you rely on when deciding whether a patient has B12 deficiency – don't forget to assess his/her symptoms, take a detailed history and perform a thorough examination.

The Methylmalonic Acid Test

Information for the Layman or Patients:

You might remember that *methylmalonic acid* accumulates in the body in the absence or low levels of B12 since this vitamin is required to change methylmalonic acid into another form that the body needs.

When you have low levels of B12 in your body, MMA (no, not Mixed Martial Arts) will begin to accumulate in your body and doctors can test its levels in your blood or urine to see if you are deficient. This test is considered better than the testing for serum B12 levels (unless the normal ranges for serum B12 are changed). If you want to know more about the normal levels, feel free to read the section on this test written for physicians.

Information for Physicians:

Methylmalonic acid can be detected both in the blood and in the urine. However, according to many studies, the urinary test is much better. Let's see why:

It is more sensitive than the test for the measurement of serum B12 levels.[104]

It is more sensitive than the serum MMA test.[105]

It is extremely specific (almost 99 %).[106]

In addition, those who have neurological impairment due to B12 deficiency excrete higher amounts than those who don't,[107] meaning this test can be used to judge whether a person is on the path of acquiring permanent neurological deficit or has already got it.[108]

Serum MMA is raised in conditions other than B12 deficiency too, such as renal insufficiency, Thyroid disease, bacterial overgrowth in the small intestine, pregnancy, hemo-concentration and sometimes because of unexplained reasons.[109]

Below are the values for both serum as well urinary methylmalonic acid that will help you distinguish the normal individuals from those who are B12 deficient -

Normal serum MMA (SMMA) ≤ 0.04 μmol/L[110] or 0.04-0.27 μmol/L
Normal Urinary MMA (uMMA) < 3.60 mmol/mol creatinine[111]

Other Tests That are Not Routinely Used or Required
Other Tests That are Not Routinely Used or Required

Usually, the serum B12 and/or MMA test along with the patients history are enough to diagnose a deficiency of B12. However, there are a few more tests you should know about that are also helpful in diagnosing this problem:

The Holotranscobalamin Test

Holotranscobalamin is the active form of B12. Usually, it makes up around 20 % of the total B12 in your serum and the Holo-TC test is designed to measure this particular amount. The normal range is 35-101 pmol/L. However, very few speciality labs carry out this test and just like the test for MMA, this test won't be required if the serum B12 levels were revised.

The Plasma Homocysteine Test
You already know a lot, (maybe even too much) about it if you read Chapter 3. Therefore, I won't obsess over it again. The normal range of Homocysteine is 2.2-13.2 μmol/L.[112]This test is rather expensive and isn't usually done on a regular basis.

The Shilling Test

This test is done to find out the cause of B12 deficiency rather than confirming whether someone has it or not since the serum B12 test and the urinary MMA test are better suited for that.

In this test, you'll be given B12 and its excretion will be checked in the urine. If abnormal results are seen, you'll have to go through a couple of stages of testing till your doctor finds out the cause of your B12 deficiency (such as stomach problems, bacterial overgrowth or pancreatic problems which could be causing a B12 deficiency).

The Cost Effectiveness of Early Screening and Treatment for B12 Deficiency
If B12 deficiency is affecting so many people, shouldn't preventive measures such as screening for early diagnosis be adopted? Many believe that this would just be a waste of money. I choose to strongly disagree, below are my reasons why:

The tests that are used to test for B12 deficiency (serum B12 levels and MMA) are much cheaper than the ones used by healthcare professionals in case of those patients whose B12 deficiency is at an advances stage. What's the point of using expensive tests such as CT-scans and MRIs at late stages (done when doctors suspect other diseases and want to rule them out) when you can easily test your patients at an early stage by using cheaper tests such as the MMA test?

Insurance companies cover the MMA test as well as the Homocysteine test – something that many physicians don't know.

If B12 deficiency is screened for AND TREATED at an early stage, the total costs of these two procedures is much less than that of treating these patients when the deficiency is severe. The reason why I mention the last stages of the deficiency over and over is that it's easier for doctors to diagnose patients when their condition has reached its last stage – a time when treatments for the multiple organ systems (that are involved due to the severe B12 deficiency) also have to be included along with the B12 therapy.

In simple terms, if detected early, the tests and the B12 therapy would cost much less as compared to late detection when numerous medications have to be given along with the multiple tests that doctors usually order.

The treatment of B12 deficiency at its early stages costs only $36 a year!

Far too many people are affected by B12 deficiency[113] and it has very rightly been called an 'epidemic' by Pacholok and Stuart in their book. Why then should we risk worsening of this condition when it is so easy to diagnose (by the help of the tests, proper history taking and thorough clinical exams) as well as treat?

Simply said, I feel as if holding back widespread preventive screening is costing us much more (both in terms of money as well the health of the general population) than diagnosing and treating B12 deficiency at later stages.

It won't be an easy job to change the standards set by health authorities in many countries. However, for all you physicians out there, it's not hard for you to begin early screening as well as treatment. There might not be defined rules or standards regarding prevention and early screening and/or diagnosis – but there aren't any rules telling you not to practice these either!

Save your patients from the horrible consequences of a severe B12 deficiency and treat them on time. When you're not sure about whether you should begin treatment or not, it's always safe to stick to a therapeutic trial since B12 isn't toxic, as mentioned earlier.

Chapter 5: How Is B12 Deficiency Treated?

General Principles

If someone has a vitamin B12 deficiency, we just give them vitamin B12. **Wrong**! Although Vitamin B12 therapy plays a vital role in the treatment of a person who is deficient in it, it is equally important to find out the cause of that person's deficiency and treat that accordingly.

Of course, if the cause is just low intake, all that's needed is regular B12 therapy, maybe even for life if the person is a strict vegetarian. The same principle applies to those who have had surgeries of the stomach or intestines and cannot absorb vitamin B12. Let's see how different causes of vitamin B12 deficiency are treated:

Those with high needs of B12:

This category includes pregnant women, children and the elderly. In these cases, since there is no 'disease' as such, only vitamin B12 needs to be given.

A) Those who have problems absorbing B12:

This group includes those people who have had surgeries of the stomach or intestine, have pancreatic problems or have pernicious anaemia. If you have had such surgeries, you will need to take vitamin B12 for the rest of your life, the same is applicable for those with pernicious anaemia.

However, those with pernicious anaemia will also require intrinsic factor and certain other drugs to suppress and control this auto-immune disease. In case of those with pancreatic problems, the pancreatic enzymes which help absorb vitamin B12 will have to be given along with B12 therapy.

B) Those who ingest toxins which lower serum B12 levels:

This includes people who have been consuming too much alcohol for a long time or been messing up with nitrous oxide. These two might make you feel like you're on top of the world for a while, but the world will soon come crashing down when they lower your B12 levels to extremely dangerous levels. Okay, maybe I'm being a little dramatic, but hey, you get the picture right? Just don't mess around with these two.

C) Those who have too many germs in their gut:

If the normal flora (which means the zillions of bacteria you harbour in your gut normally) overgrow, they'll start eating up your B12. All that will be needed then is a course of antibiotics along with some B12 therapy and you'll be as good as new, well at least in case of B12!

D) Those who are taking medications that interfere with B12 levels:

Like I mentioned in chapter 2, drugs such as Metformin lowers B12 levels. Such drugs might have to be replaced or concomitant B12 therapy could be initiated to keep the patient from having a B12 deficiency.

What are the Various Forms of Vitamin B12?
What are the Various Forms of Vitamin B12?

You might recall a particularly bland and boring part of chapter 2 where I somewhat forcefully bombarded you with the various forms of the different forms of vitamin B12 – those weird chemical names such as *hydroxycobalamin* or *cyanocobalamin*.

Well, I admit that information is pretty boring if you don't know what it's used for. That part was about the chemical basics. Here's the scoop:

> There are three types or forms of vitamin B12: *Cyanocobalamin, Hydroxycobalamin, Adenosylcobalamin* and *Methylcobalamin*.

> *Adenosylcobalamin* and *Methylcobalamin* are the only two forms present in the human body – the former is present within your blood and is readily to all the cells that need it whereas the latter is present in tiny parts of your cells, called mitochondria which are the energy production centres of all cells.

How is that information helpful to us?[114]

Injections, tablets, patches, sprays – those are the various preparations available as a vitamin B12 therapy. These preparations contain any one of those 4 forms listed above. We have to decide what the best form of B12[115] is so that we get maximum results with our B12 therapy.

So which form is the best then? Here's what you need to know -

Cyanocobalamin is the most stubborn form – that's because in this type, the B12 is bound to a cyanide group which won't let B12 get free that easily. Yes, it does protect B12 from extreme conditions (such as high temperature, etc) but it doesn't let the body free up the B12 that's bound to it. That's not all. There's another reason why we shouldn't like this form of B12 – that's the fact that cyanocobalamin is excreted by the kidneys, as if it's some toxin bound to B12 (which is one of B12's functions, remember?). So of course, none of us like getting our B12 flushed out whenever we eat it with the intent to replenish our stores.

Since the body uses *methylcobalamin* and *adenosylcobalamin*, these forms are the best when it comes to what form of B12 you should take.

The form *hydroxycobalamin* can also be used by your body after it's converted to *methylcobalamin*, however it's slightly more expensive and hard to manufacture.

So that makes it pretty clear that you should take any form of B12, apart from *cyanocobalamin*. Again, *hydroxycobalamin* is expensive, so you can take any of the other two.

What Are The Various Preparations of Vitamin B12?
What Are The Various Preparations of Vitamin B12?

When you need a vitamin therapy for a deficiency or just regular supplementation (in case you're a vegan, have had stomach surgery, etc) you'll obviously want to know what various methods of treatment or supplementation are available.

Without further ado, here's the list along with some brief information to help you decide what you want to use (In consultation with your doctor because I haven't included all the information here, such as the dosage, so make sure you get a consultation with a specialist or your physician regarding what form and dosage of B12 you need since different people need different amounts[116]:

Oral Forms of Vitamin B12

Liquid B12 and Oral Tablets (The ones you swallow):

Most dietary supplements contain B12 but those which contain only B12 or vitamins B6, B9 and B12 are also available.

Pros: Easily available (over-the-counter), relatively inexpensive, easy to administer.

Cons: Most supplements contain *cyanocobalamin.*[117]

Supplements contain large amounts of B12 but very little of this is absorbed. If you take a supplement with 500 mcg of B12, only about 10 mcg will be absorbed.[118] That's because no matter how much B12 you take, the amount of intrinsic factor in your stomach is produced to a limited extent.[119] The extra B12 isn't absorbed.

Many patients recover much sooner with injections as compared to when they are given tablets. Therefore, these tablets are only suitable for use when you're a vegetarian or just want to make sure you're getting enough B12.

Sublingual Tablets (the ones you place under your tongue):

You might come across ads of sublingual B12 tablets (the ones you place under your tongue) that claim this form is better than the tablet that you can swallow. There is no evidence to support such claims[120] so whether you're taking oral or sublingual tablets, the results will be the same![121]

Pros: Same as the ones for oral tablets, however sublingual ones are somewhat cheaper.

Cons: Same as that for the oral tablets.

Oral Sprays:

Pros: Gets a very high amount of B12 into your blood, more than the supplemental form does.[122]

Cons: This form is expensive.

Vitamin B12 Injections

Pros:

Do not depend on Intrinsic Factor so whatever is administered goes directly into the blood and the excess is flushed out in the urine.

Large doses can be given in one injection, eliminating the need for you take them daily or 2-3 times a week, which is the case with tablets.

Are not expensive.

You can get the effective Methylcobalamin form.

Cons:

Are not available over-the-counter (though you can buy them from the link above)

Are prescribed for states of deficiency.[123]

You would need to learn how to inject yourself or have someone do it for you.

The area where you inject yourself might hurt.

Vitamin B12 Nasal Spray

Pros:

Contains amounts comparable to those present in injections.

No need to use needles.

You don't have to learn how to use this form of B12, as is the case with B12 shots/injections.

Are available over-the-counter as well as by prescription.

Cons:

Nasal sprays are expensive. Damn.

Some contain *cyanocobalamin*.

Vitamin B12 Nasal Gel

Pros:

An excellent alternative for those patients of B12 deficiency who do not want to use injections.[124]

Is very effective in increasing the B12 levels in your blood.[125]

Cons:

Usually available by prescription only.

Slightly expensive.

Vitamin B12 Patches:

Pros:

Very easy to use.

No need for multiple doses, you only need to wear it once a week for a total period of 24 hours.

Is an excellent and efficient way of delivering B12 to your body, some call it the best preparation of B12.

It can easily be ordered online.

It doesn't cost much because you wear it just once a week.

Cons:

Some people might experience a skin reaction, therefore look out for that when you wear the patch.

A few things you need to know before you begin any of the above medications:

Inform your doctor if you have any of the following conditions (in case he doesn't ask about it himself):

If you're trying to conceive or are pregnant.

If you're breastfeeding.

If you're allergic to cobalamin or any of its forms.

If you have folic acid deficiency or *megaloblastic anaemia*.

If you have nasal congestion (due to an infection or allergies) in case you're opting for any of the nasal form of B12 preparations.

If you're taking any medications so that your doctor can decide whether these should be changed due to interaction with B12, etc.

Note: *Cut down your intake of Alcohol to achieve the best results of a B12 therapy.*

Side Effects of B12 Therapy/Supplementation

Medications have side effects so doesn't B12 have any? Not really – unless you're that one rare person out of zillions of people who might be allergic to it. Here are some side effects that have been observed, albeit very uncommonly, with B12 therapy:

The EXTREMELY rare ones: Allergic reactions, wheezing, chest tightness and pain, dizziness, fever, itching. (Report to your doctor as soon as you get any of side effects!)

The unlikely ones (but slightly more common than the rare ones): Nausea, diarhea, headaches (Usually get better with time but if they bother you too much, contact your physician).

Is B12 Toxic in High Doses

I think you already know the answer to this one! If not, I'll repeat what I've said a couple of times earlier in the previous chapters – B12 is perfectly safe in high doses, no associated toxicity whatsoever.

I have never seen any case of an over-B12'd person. Until and if that black swan comes, it is perfectly reasonable to assume high doses are safe.

Chapter 6: The Misdiagnosis of B12 Deficiency

Misdiagnosis Oversight

When I was making a list of all the diseases or conditions that could possibly mimic B12 deficiency, I started looking online and read up everything I could find which was appropriate to my search queries. I came across one particular post that made me stop what I was looking for, only to find myself wondering how life could get upside down within a matter of days or weeks without leaving us with any hope of ever getting better.

No, it wasn't cancer that I read about. It wasn't even a stroke that left someone permanently paralysed – it was worse. Someone had been diagnosed with end stage kidney failure when she most probably had a vitamin B12 deficiency. She had listed her symptoms to get the opinion of an expert.[126]

The symptoms that had been described were hair loss, weight loss, appetite changes, sweating, rashes on the sides of the face and the neck, and vertigo.

In addition, this particular person had low grade fevers, low sugar levels, low blood pressure and had donated one of her kidneys to her mother (due to which doctors couldn't biopsy her kidney to diagnose what disease had caused her kidneys to fail).

If you look at those symptoms, you know there's something very familiar about them. Here's the shocker: this patient was TOLD that she has a B12 deficiency. That particular fact made it hard for me to decide what my reaction should be. Apart from shock, there was literally nothing else I could feel.

Have our medical skills, years of research and state-of-the-art facilities been of no use at all? Why can't we diagnose, detect and treat something that is right in front of us? To all the doctors, medical students and nurses out there – that's a thought to ponder upon.

I'm sure some of you are thinking 'how can you be so sure that it was

B12 deficiency? There's so many conditions that could present with similar symptoms.' In reply I'd like to say just this: If B12 isn't toxic, why don't we begin therapeutic trials in those who COULD have it? Wouldn't we be criminals if we ignored such an easily treatable condition based on only the fact that we're not sure if this is what's causing the problems, when the treatment does no harm at all? Would you let someone die even when you knew they had a very fat chance of surviving with a harmless therapeutic trial?

Getting back to the symptoms listed above – the patient had asked whether she had lupus (an autoimmune disease, which can also cause similar problems). The expert who answered the question implied it most probably is a B12 deficiency; she had suffered from it themselves.

What Diseases Can Mimic B12 Deficiency?

What Diseases Can Mimic B12 Deficiency

From the above story, it's very obvious that knowing the conditions that can have similar symptoms to that of a B12 deficiency is equally important as knowing how B12 deficiency affects your body. Let's go through short descriptions of all these conditions:

Conditions of the Gastrointestinal Tract

Irritable Bowel Syndrome

This is a condition somewhat poorly misunderstood by doctors when it comes to how and why it begins and affects certain individuals. It is characterised by bouts of diarrhoea or constipation or both. In addition, vague symptoms such as indigestion, bloating, abdominal pain, etc are also felt.

These symptoms are very real but there's literally no cause within the body that points at why the patient has these issues. You might remember from chapter 3 that B12 deficiency affects your gastrointestinal tract (because these cells are rapidly growing) and causes similar vague symptoms.

Crohn's Disease

This is an autoimmune disease in which the lining of the GIT is damaged and it results in diarrhoea, abdominal pain, blood in stools, indigestion, malabsorption, etc – all very similar to those caused by a B12 deficiency.

Conditions of the Nervous System

Multiple Sclerosis

Another auto-immune condition, this disease eventually rips of the myelin sheaths off of your nerves, very much like B12 deficiency does. Needless to say, it causes very similar symptoms. This disease affects many people, usually in their 20's and 30's, comes all of a sudden in attacks with completely symptomless periods. It causes walking problems, deterioration of vision, failure to balance oneself, etc – pretty much all the same as those caused by B12 deficiency.

Interestingly, many people who have MS also have a B12 deficiency.[127]

Dementia & Alzheimer's Disease

As I mentioned in Chapter 3, when your brain is affected by B12 deficiency, you could develop symptoms such as memory loss and failure to concentrate – something called dementia. Alzheimer's also closely mimics B12 deficiency, owing to its manifestations of a decreased short term memory, irritability, and personality changes.

Psychiatric Disorders

B12 deficiency causes emotional imbalance and behavioural changes, as you already know after having read chapter 3. The symptoms of depression, personality changes, irritability, confusion, delirium, mania, hallucinations and psychosis can all fit into almost any psychiatric condition.

From clinical depression and psychotic attacks to autism spectrum disorder[128], B12 deficiency could present with almost any psychiatric problem. Therefore, it HAS to be included in the valid differential diagnoses of mental disorders.

Diabetic Neuropathy

Diabetes causes damage to your nerves, causes tingling and sensations of pins and needles (these are the ones most commonly seen but just about any nerve can be affected causing symptoms related to the nerve involved.

For example, if diabetes affects the nerve that supplies the muscles of your eyes, you'll get double vision and problems in moving your eyes). Again, B12 deficiency could do that too.

Developmental Delay in Children

If you have been told that your child will not develop as fast as other children his/her child and might have learning disabilities, there's a chance that he/she might be suffering from a B12 deficiency (as mentioned in chapter 3). Infants of strict vegetarian mothers are at the greatest risk.

If you're one of them, do not forget to supplement your diet with B12 since your child's nervous system is in the stages of development and anything going wrong at this time could cause permanent damage.

Parkinson's Disease

Parkinson's disease causes problems in normal daily activities such as buttoning up one's shirt, walking, etc – basically impairing your coordinated movements. When B12 deficiency affects your nervous system, it can cause very similar symptoms.

Optic Neuritis

This is a condition that results in the inflammation of the nerve that processes whatever you see – the optic nerve. It causes visual problems due to destruction of the nerve fibres in the eye that 'perceive' what you see.

If left untreated, eventually all fibres will degenerate, leaving a person blind. Since B12 deficiency damages the myelin sheaths of all nerves, the optic nerve can also be affected. Before this treatable disorder blinds you, get your B12 levels checked.

Vertigo

When your vestibular nerve (a nerve that is responsible for the maintenance of balance by sensing signals from tiny, special organs within your ears) is damaged, you will have balance problems and the world around you will seem to be spinning – that's vertigo.

There are numerous causes of that, including a B12 deficiency. Get your B12 levels checked before you end up damaging nerves permanently. Ouch.

Restless Legs Syndrome

This is a condition in which you'll feel weird tingly sensations creeping up your legs, making you shake your legs to get rid of them. When low B12 levels damage your nerves, you can definitely feel such crazy things.

There are other causes of this problem too but B12 deficiency is one of them which is why you should get your B12 levels checked if you're experiencing similar problems.

Cardiovascular and Haematological Disorders

Folate Deficiency

Folate and B12 work together for the synthesis of DNA for red blood cells in the bone marrow (in addition to other cells) which is why their deficiency shows up as megaloblastic anaemia (in which the red blood cells are large and immature, with decreased lifespans).

The symptoms of anaemia (no matter what the cause) are the same and in this case, the blood smear test will show the same type of large red blood cells which is why you might get diagnosed with folate deficiency when you're actually suffering from B12 deficiency.

Treatment with folate will be dangerous because it will mask the anaemia but the nervous system will continue to get damaged due to the low B12 levels. You will eventually suffer from permanent neurological injury if you remain untreated for B12 deficiency and don't notice your symptoms in time.

Heart Disease & Strokes

Since low B12 causes high homocysteine levels (which leads to atherosclerosis or thickening of your blood vessels), you might suffer from heart attack and heart failure, having all the symptoms of heart disease. In addition, you might have strokes and get permanent damage to your brain.

Infertility, PMS & PMDD

As mentioned in chapter 3, low B12 levels have been linked with infertility in men as well as women along with recurrent miscarriages.

Some couples might be diagnosed to have 'idiopathic' infertility (where the cause isn't known) where one of them might be suffering from a B12 deficiency.

In addition, pre-menstrual syndrome and pre-menstrual distress disorder have both been associated with low B12 levels.

You might not need those antidepressants to treat these annoying conditions because B12 deficiency is a valid differential diagnosis. B12 shots could be the cure!

Hypothyroidism

Depression, lethargy, excessive somnolence (sleeping too much), etc – those are the symptoms of hypothyroidism. But even low B12 levels can cause the same problems, as you already know. In addition, those who have pernicious anaemia are at higher risk of getting hypothyroidism – they're linked both ways!

Miscellaneous Disorders

Systemic Lupus Erythmatosus

This is an auto-immune condition which can cause numerous symptoms, some of which include fatigue, muscular pain, confusion, joint pain, skin rashes, etc. Many of these are also present in B12 deficient patients.

Interestingly, the story at the beginning of this chapter was from a post by a patient whose question was "Do I have Lupus?" The expert had strongly suspected pernicious Anaemia, a cause of B12 deficiency.

Chronic Fatigue Syndrome

As its name implies, this condition causes fatigue, dull pains and feeling tired all the time despite getting enough sleep. B12 deficiency causes the same, remember?

Fibromyalgia

This disorder isn't very well-understood. Patients who have this problem experience severe pain in certain areas of the body, called 'pain points.' The pain is excruciating and unbearable for some and it is said that it is a result of the brain over-reacting to painful stimuli. Other symptoms include confusion, trouble concentrating, dizziness, depression, sleeping problems, etc. These should sounds very familiar by now.

Therefore, you can see that numerous conditions present with symptoms very similar to those caused by B12 deficiency. In addition to keeping patients untreated and at risk for permanent damage to their body, doctors cause loss of extremely large amounts of money[129] when they misdiagnose these disorders. Most of these conditions need chronic therapy by expensive drugs and sometimes even hospitalization. Misdiagnosis is thus costing us our health as well large sums of money.

Helpful Resources

Vitamin B12 Deficiency Support Group (Charity) – a real, no-fluff resource for B12 deficiency. The website is based on the latest research, and these guys know what they're talking about.

www.b12d.org

TrimNutrition – a great provider of various nutritional supplements. They have the Methylcobalamin shots I have recommended along the book. You'll have to book a meeting with them though, B12 injections are illegal to sell in the U.S now without a face-to-face doctor consultation.

TrimNutrition.com

NutritionData – a great resource for checking the nutritional values of every possible food.

NutritionData.com

Lastly,

I'd like to thank **Dr. Hugo Minney** from the "B12 Deficiency Support Group" who provided us with some research papers, very valuable information, and also gave us the protocol for the diagnosis of B12 deficiency which was made by **Dr. Joseph Chandy** who I'd like to thank as well for the 'indirect' help. Doctors really NEED this protocol, and we'll try to make sure it's being used more.

In addition, I want to thank *Regev Elya* (architect and editor of this book) and my parents, *Ghazanfar Ali Khan* and *Samina Ali Khan*, for the constant support – I almost gave up in the middle but you guys told me to keep going. That's more valuable to me than any other kind of help.

Final Words and Bonus Gifts

Hey guys! Regev here again.

To show my appreciation to you, I've created two nice PDFs you can print and use. The first one is a fridge-list containing the best foods containing vitamin B12. The other list is a checklist with all the various symptoms of a B12 deficiency. Print them both, put them on your fridge and shall your health prosper.

Here are the links:

http://freshbeetle.com/foods.pdf

http://freshbeetle.com/symptoms.pdf

I hope the book helped you understand B12-deficiency a little bit better. When I first started this project, I never imagined it will take us so much time to implement, but I'm very happy with the final result, and I hope you too.

We spent a lot of time and effort creating this book, and I would really appreciate if you would respect us and not share or distribute the book to anyone else without our permission. Lots of gooooooood karma if you help us and report if you ever come across pirated copies.

Aight Regev! What Should I Do Next?

Help spread the word by leaving a 5-star review if you think this book is helpful. Good reviews help us to reach more people and help. Bonus love points if you go the extra mile and add some text to your review.

Take good care of yourself, I'm all hope that through this book, B12 deficiency will never be an issue for you.

---

[1] *McBride, J., 2000, B12 Deficiency May Be More Widespread Than Thought.*

[2] *Stabler, S.P., Allen, R.H., 2004, Vitamin B12 Deficiency as a Worldwide Problem, Annual Review of Nutrition, V : 24, P: 299-326.*

[3] Marsh, K., Zeuschner, C., Saunders, A., 2012, Health Implications of a Vegetarian Diet, American Journal of Lifestyle Medicine, V :6, P : 250-267.

[4] Oiso, T., 1975, . Incidence of Stomach Cancer and Its Relation to Dietary Habits and Nutrition in Japan between 1900 and 1975, Cancer Res , V: 35; P: 3254.

[5] Smith, D.A. & Refsum,H.,2009, Vitamin B-12 and cognition in the elderly, American Journal of Clinical Nutrition, V:2, P: 707S-711.

[6] Abyad A, 2002, Prevalence of vitamin B12 deficiency among demented patients and cognitive recovery with cobalamin replacement, The Journal of Nutrition, Health & Aging, V : 6(4), P: 254-60.

[7] "Dietary Supplement Fact Sheet: Vitamin B12". National Institutes of Health: Office of Dietary Supplements. http://dietary-supplements.info.nih.gov/ factsheets/vitaminb12.asp. Retrieved June 2,2012.

[8] Institute of Medicine. Food and Nutrition Board. Dietary Reference Intakes: Thiamin, Riboflavin, Niacin, Vitamin B6, Folate, Vitamin B12, Pantothenic Acid, Biotin, and Choline. Washington, DC: National Academy Press, 1998

[9] Fischbach F. A Manual of Laboratory & Diagnostic Tests, 6th Ed. Philadelphia, PA: Lippincott Williams & Wilkins; 2000.

[10] Stabler,S.P. Screening the older population for cobalamin (vitamin B12) deficiency. J am Geriatr Soc. 1995 Nov; 43 (11):1290-1297.

[11] Shahar,A.,Feuglin,L.,Shahar, D.R.,Levy,S., and Seligsohn,U High Prevalence and impact of subnormal serum vitamin B12 levels in Israeli elders admitted to a geriatric hospital. Journal of Nutrition, Health and Aging (2001) 5:124-7

[12] Pennypacker, L.C., Allen, R.H.,Kelly J.P., et al. High Prevalence of cobalamin deficiency in elderly outpatients. J Am Geriatr Soc. 1992 Dec; 40(12):1197-1204.

[13] Dharmajan, T.S.,Adiga, G.U.,Norkus,E.P. Vitamin B12 deficiency. Recognising subtle symptoms in older adults. Geriatrics 2003;58:30-8.

[14] U.S. Department of Agriculture, Agricultural Research Service. 2011. USDA

National Nutrient Database for Standard Reference, Release 24. Nutrient Data Laboratory Home Page, http://www.ars.usda.gov/ba/bhnrc/ndl.

[15] Walsh, Stephen (2003). Plant Based Nutrition and Health. The Vegan Society. ISBN 0-907337-279.

[16] Davis, Brenda and Vesanto Melina (2000). Becoming Vegan. Book Publishing Company. ISBN 1-57067-103-6.

[17] Walsh, Stephen, RD. "Vegan Society B12 factsheet". Vegan Society.

[18] http://www.vegansociety.com/food/nutrition/b12/. Retrieved 2012-06-02.

[19] von Schenck U, Bender-Gotze C, Koletzko B. Persistence of neurological damage induced by dietary vitamin B12 deficiency in infancy. Arch Dis Childhood 1997;77:137-9.

[20] Kaiser L, Allen LH. Position of the American Dietetic Association: nutrition and lifestyle for a healthy pregnancy outcome. J Am Diet Assoc 2008;108:553-61.

[21] Sumner AE, Chin MM, Abraham JL, Gerry GT, Allen RH, Stabler SP. Elevated methylmalonic acid and total homocysteine levels show high prevalence of vitamin B12 deficiency after gastric surgery. Ann Intern Med 1996;124:469-76.

[22] Doscherholmen A, Swaim WR. Impaired assimilation of egg Co 57 vitamin B 12 in patients with hypochlorhydria and achlorhydria and after gastric resection. Gastroenterology 1973;64:913-9.

[23] Brolin RE, Gorman JH, Gorman RC, Petschenik A J, Bradley L J, Kenler H A, et al. Are vitamin B12 and folate deficiency clinically important after roux-en-Y gastric bypass? J Gastrointest Surg 1998;2:436-42.

[24] Cordingley FT, Crawford GP (1986). "Giardia infection causes vitamin B12 deficiency". Aust N Z J Med 16 (1): 78–9.

[25] Burnham TH,Drug Facts and Comparisons. St. Louis, MO: Facts and Comparisons,2001.

[26] McEvoy GK,American Hospital Formulary Service Drug Information. Bethesda, MD: American Society of Health-System Pharmacists,2001.

[27] Bratman S.,The Natural Pharmacist – Drug Herb Interactions Bible.Roseville, CA:Prima Publishing,2001.

[28] Liu KW, Dai LK, Jean W. Metformin-related vitamin B12 deficiency. Age Ageing 2006;35:200-1.

[29] Buvat DR. Use of metformin is a cause of vitamin B12 deficiency. Am Fam Physician 2004;69:264.

[30] de Jager J, Kooy A, Lehert P, Wulffelé MG, van der Kolk J, Bets D, Verburg J, Donker AJ, Stehouwer CD. Long term treatment with metformin in patients with type 2 diabetes and risk of vitamin B-12 deficiency: randomised placebo controlled trial. BMJ. 2010 May 20;340:c2181.

[31] Oh R, Brown DL. Use of metformin is a cause of vitamin B12 deficiency. Author Reply Am Fam Physician 2004;69:264, 266.

[32] Valuck RJ, Ruscin JM. A case-control study on adverse effects: H2 blocker or proton pump inhibitor use and risk of vitamin B12 deficiency in older adults. J Clin Epidemiol 2004;57:422-8.

[33] Force RW, Nahata MC. Effect of histamine H2-receptor antagonists on vitamin B12 absorption. Ann Pharmacother 1992;26:1283-6.

[34] Bradford GS and Taylor CT. Omeprazole and vitamin B12 deficiency. Ann Pharmacother 1999;33:641-3.

[35] Howden CW. Vitamin B12 levels during prolonged treatment with proton pump inhibitors. J Clin Gastroenterol 2000;30:29-33.

[36] Den Elzen WP, Groeneveld Y, De Ruijter W, Souverijn JH, Le Cessie S, Assendelft WJ, et al. Long-term use of proton pump inhibitors (PPIs) and vitamin B12 status in elderly individuals. Aliment Pharmacol Ther 2008;27:491-7.

[37] Ruscin JM, Page RL 2nd, Valuck RJ. Vitamin B(12) deficiency associated with histamine(2)-receptor antagonists and a proton-pump inhibitor. Ann Pharmacother 2002;36:812-6.

[38] Termanini B, Gibril F, Sutliff VE, Yu F, Venzon DJ, Jensen RT. Effect of long-term gastric acid suppressive therapy on serum vitamin B12 levels in patients with Zollinger-Ellison syndrome. Am J Med 1998;104:422-30.

[39] Lindenbaum J & Liber C. S. Alcohol-induced Malabsorption of Vitamin B12 in Man, Nature 1969; 224, 806

[40] Carmel R. Prevalence of undiagnosed pernicious anemia in the elderly. Arch Intern Med 1996;156:1097-100.

[41] Huritz A, Brady DA, Schaal SE, Samloff IM, Dedon J, Ruhl CE. Gastric acidity in older adults. J Am Med Assoc 1997;278:659-62.

[42] Andrews GR, Haneman B, Arnold BJ, Booth JC, Taylor K. Atrophic gastritis in the aged. Aust Ann Med 1967;16:230-5.

[43] Johnsen R, Bernersen B, Straume B, Forder OH, Bostad L, Burhol PG. Prevalence of endoscopic and histological findings in subjects with and without dyspepsia. Br Med J 1991;302:749-52.

[44] Krasinski SD, Russell R, Samloff IM, Jacob RA, Dalal GE, McGandy RB, et al. Fundic atrophic gastritis in an elderly population: Effect on hemoglobin and several serum nutritional indicators. J Am Geriatr Soc 1986;34:800-6.

[45] www.b12d.org/

[46] www.b12d.org

[47] B, Shane; Stokstad, E L R (1985). Vitamin B12-Folate Interrelationships. Ann. Rev. Nutr 5: 115–41.

[48] Anatol Dowzenko Clinical Neurology ISBN 83-200-1197-3, p. 451

[49] Dietrich-Muszalska A, Malinowska J, Olas B, et al. (May 2012). The oxidative stress may be induced by the elevated homocysteine in schizophrenic patients. Neurochem. Res. 37 (5): 1057–62.

[50] Kivipelto M, Annerbo S, Hultdin J, et al. (July 2009). Homocysteine and holo-transcobalamin and the risk of dementia and Alzheimers disease: a prospective study. European Journal of Neurology 16 (7): 808–13.

[51] Sethi NK, Robilotti E, Sadan Y (2005). Neurological Manifestations Of Vitamin B-12 Deficiency. The Internet Journal of Nutrition and Wellness 2 (1).

[52] Masalha R, Chudakov B, Muhamad M, Rudoy I, Volkov I, Wirguin I (2001). Cobalamin-responsive psychosis as the sole manifestation of vitamin B12 deficiency. Israeli Medical Association Journal 3: 701–703.

[53] http://www.nlm.nih.gov/medlineplus/ency/article/000569.htm

[54] Kageyama M, Hiraoka M, Kagawa Y (October 2008). Relationship between genetic polymorphism, serum folate and homocysteine in Alzheimer's disease. Asia-Pacific Journal of Public Health 20 Suppl: 111–7.

[55] Siuda J, Gorzkowska A, Patalong-Ogiewa M, et al. (2009). From mild cognitive impairment to Alzheimer's disease - influence of homocysteine, vitamin B12 and folate on cognition over time: results from one-year follow-up. Neurologia I Neurochirurgia Polska 43 (4): 321–9.

[56] Vogiatzoglou A, Refsum H, Johnston C, Smith S.M., Bradley K.M, de Jager C, Budge M.M. and Smith A.D, Vitamin B12 status and rate of brain volume loss in community-dwelling elderly, Neurology 2008;71 (11)826-832

[57] Sachdev P.S., Valenzuela M.,Wang X.L., Looi J. C.L., Brodaty H., Relationship between plasma homocysteine levels and brain atrophy in healthy elderly individuals, Neurology 2002; 58 (10):1539-1541

[58] .Baldewicz TT, Goodkin K, Blaney NT, Shor-Posner G, Kumar M, Wilkie FL, Baum MK, Eisdorfer C. Cobalamin level is related to self-reported and clinically rated mood and to syndromal depression in bereaved HIV-1+ and HIV-1- homosexual men. J Psychosom Res. 2000;48177- 185

[59] Coppen A.,Christina Bolander-Gouaille C.,Treatment of depression: time to consider folic acid and vitamin B12,J Psychopharmacol January 2005; 19(1) 59-65.

[60] Tiemeier H, Van Tuijl HR, Hofman A, Meijer J, Kiliaan AJ, Breteler MM. Vitamin B12, folate, and homocysteine in depression: the Rotterdam Study. Am J Psychiatry. 2002;1592099- 2101

[61] Fava M, Borus JS, Alpert JE, Nierenberg AA, Rosenbaum JF, Bottiglieri T. Folate, vitamin B12, and homocysteine in major depressive disorder. Am J Psychiatry. 1997;154426- 428

[62] Brenda W.J.H. Penninx B.W.H., Guralnik J.M., Ferrucci L., Fried L.P.,Allen R.H., Stabler S.P., Vitamin B12 Deficiency and Depression in Physically Disabled Older Women: Epidemiologic Evidence From the Women's Health and Aging Study,Am J Psychiatry 2000;157:715-721.

[63] Selhub J, Bagley LC, Miller J, Rosenberg IH. B vitamins, homocysteine,

and neurocognitive function in the elderly. Am J Clin Nutr. 2000;71 suppl614S-620S

[64] *Clarke R, Smith AD, Jobst KA, Refsum H, Sutton L, Ueland PM. Folate, vitamin B12, and serum total homocysteine levels in confirmed Alzheimer disease. Arch Neurol. 1998;551449- 1455*

[65] *Sonja A. Rasmussen, Paul M. Fernhoff, Kelley S. Scanlon,Vitamin B12 deficiency in children and adolescents,The Journal of Pediatrics,January 2001;138 (1)Pages 10-17.*

[66] *Grahama S.M., Arvelaa O.M., Wise G. A,Long-term neurologic consequences of nutritional vitamin B12 deficiency in infants,The Journal of Paediatrics,November 1992;121(5), Part 1, p.710–714*

[67] *Miller JW, Nadeau MR, Smith D and Selhub J (1994). "Vitamin B-6 deficiency vs folate deficiency: comparison of responses to methionine loading in rats". American Journal of Clinical Nutrition 59 (5): 1033–1039.*

[68] *Gallai V, Caso V, et al. Mild hyperhomocyst(e)inemia: a possible risk factor for cervical artery dissection. Stroke. 2001;32:714-718.*

[69] *Papatheodorou L, Weiss N. Vascular oxidant stress and inflammation in hyperhomocysteinemia. Antioxid Redox Signal. 2007;9:1941-1958.*

[70] *Hofmann MA, Lalla E, et al. Hyperhomocysteinemia enhances vascular inflammation and accelerates atherosclerosis in a murine model. J Clin Invest. 2001;107:675-683.*

[71] *Osanai T, Fujiwara N, et al. Novel pro-atherogenic molecule coupling factor 6 is elevated in patients with stroke: a possible linkage to homocysteine. Ann Med. 2010;42:79-86.*

[72] *Zeng X, Dai J, et al. Homocysteine mediated expression and secretion of monocyte chemoattractant protein- I and Interleukin-8 in human monocytes. Circ Res. 2003;93:311-320.*

[73] *"B vitamins do not protect hearts". BBC News (BBC). September 6, 2005.*

[74] *Saposnik G, Ray JG, et al, Heart Outcomes Prevention Evaluation 2 Investigators. Homocysteine-lowering therapy and stroke risk, severity, and disability: additional findings from the HOPE 2 trial. Stroke.*

2009;40:1365-1372.

[75] *Coen DA Stehouwer, Coen van Guldener (2001). Homocysteine-lowering treatment: an overview. Expert Opinion on Pharmacotherapy 2 (9): 1449–1460.*

[76] *Moschiano F, D'Amico D, et al. Homocysteine plasma levels in patients with migraine with aura. Neurol Sci. 2008;29 Suppl 1:S173-S175.*

[77] *Hamed SA. The vascular risk associations with migraine: relation to migraine susceptibility and progression. Atherosclerosis. 2009;205:15-22.*

[78] *Lea R, Colson N, et al. The effects of vitamin supplementation and MTHFR (C677T) genotype on homocysteine-lowering and migraine disability. Pharmacogenet Genomics. 2009;19:422-428.*

[79] *Kurth T, Ridker PM, et al. Migraine and biomarkers of cardiovascular disease in women. Cephalalgia. 2008;28:49-56.*

[80] *Rochtchina E, Wang JJ, et al. Elevated serum homocysteine, low serum vitamin B12, folate, and age-related macular degeneration: the Blue Mountains Eye Study. Am J Ophthalmol. 2007;143:344-346.*

[81] *Christen WG, Glynn RJ, et al. Folic acid, pyridoxine, and cyanocobalamin combination treatment and age-related macular degeneration in women: the Women's Antioxidant and Folic Acid Cardiovascular Study. Arch Intern Med. 2009;169:335-341.*

[82] *TAMURA, J.,KUBOTA, K.,MURAKAMI, H.,SAWAMURA, M.,MATSUSHIMA, T.,TAMURA, T.,SAITOH, T.,KURABAYSHI, H.,NARUSE, T.,Immunomodulation by vitamin B12: augmentation of CD8+ T lymphocytes and natural killer (NK) cell activity in vitamin B12-deficient patients by methyl-B12 treatment,Clinical & Experimental Immunology,2009; 116(1): 28-32*

[83] *Rosane N-A,Nabriski D. A. ; Braverman L. E., Shilo L., Eliahu W., Tamar R., Menachem S., Louis S.,Prevalence and Evaluation of B12 Deficiency in Patients with Autoimmune Thyroid Disease,American Journal of the Medical Sciences, 2006;332(3):119-122*

[84] *Perros, P.,Singh, R. K.,Ludlam, C. A.,Frier, B. M.,Prevalence of pernicious anaemia in patients with Type 1 diabetes mellitus and autoimmune thyroid*

disease,Diabetic Medicine,2000;17(10):749-751.

[85] Meecham J, Jones E.W, Addison's Disease and Addisonian Anaemia, The Lancet,1967;289(7489):535-538

[86] Bennett M.,Vitamin B12 deficiency, infertility and recurrent fetal loss,J Reprod Med. 2001 Mar;46(3):209-12.

[87] Sanfilippo JS, Liu YK.,Vitamin B12 deficiency and infertility: report of a case,Int J Fertil. 1991 Jan-Feb;36(1):36-8.

[88] Fenech M.,The role of folic acid and VitaminB12 in genomic stability of human cells,Mutation Research/Fundamental and Molecular Mechanisms of Mutagenesis,2001;475:(1–2)57–67.

[89] Kondo, H; Osborne, M; Kolhouse, J; Allen, R; Podell, E R; Utley, C S; Abrams, R S; Allen, R H (May 1981). Nitrous oxide has multiple deleterious effects on cobalamin metabolism and causes decreases in activities of both mammalian cobalamin-dependent enzymes in rats. The Journal of Clinical Investigation (The American Society For Clinical Investigation) 67 (5): 1270–1283.

[90] Kaiser L, Allen LH. Position of the American Dietetic Association: nutrition and lifestyle for a healthy pregnancy outcome. J Am Diet Assoc 2008;108:553-61.

[91] Institute of Medicine. Food and Nutrition Board. Dietary Reference Intakes: Thiamin, Riboflavin, Niacin, Vitamin B6, Folate, Vitamin B12, Pantothenic Acid, Biotin, and Choline. Washington, DC: National Academy Press, 1998

[92] von Schenck U, Bender-Gotze C, Koletzko B. Persistence of neurological damage induced by dietary vitamin B12 deficiency in infancy. Arch Dis Childhood 1997;77:137-9.

[93] Sklar R.,Nutritional Vitamin B12 Deficiency in a Breast-fed Infant of a Vegan-diet Mother,Clin Pediatr,1986; 25:(4) 219-221.

[94] Lukaski HC. Vitamin and mineral status: effects on physical performance. Nutrition 2004;20:632-44.

[95] Institute of Medicine. Food and Nutrition Board. Dietary Reference Intakes: Thiamin, Riboflavin, Niacin, Vitamin B6, Folate, Vitamin B12,

Pantothenic Acid, Biotin, and Choline. Washington, DC: National Academy Press, 1998

[96] *Lonn E, Yusuf S, Arnold MJ, Sheridan P, Pogue J, Micks M, et al. Homocysteine lowering with folic acid and B vitamins in vascular disease. N Engl J Med. 2006;354:1567-77.*

[97] *Bonaa KH, Njolstad I, Ueland PM, Schirmer H, Tverdal A, Steigen T, et al. Homocysteine lowering and cardiovascular events after acute myocardial infarction. N Engl J Med 2006;354:1578-88.*

[98] *Tucker KL, Rich S, Rosenberg I, Jacques P, Dallal G, Wilson WF, et al. Plasma vitamin B12 concentrations relate to intake source in the Framingham Offspring Study. Am J Clin Nutr 2000;71:514-22.*

[99] *Fischbach F. A Manual of Laboratory & Diagnostic Tests, 6th Ed. Philadelphia, PA: Lippincott Williams & Wilkins; 2000.*

[100] *Pacholok S.M.& Stuart J.J, An Invisible Epidemic,In:Could it be B12? 2nd ed. California: Quill Driver Books;2011, p 1-26.*

[101] *VanTiggelen,C.J.M,et al.Assessment of vitamin-B12 status in CSF,American Journal of Psychiatry ,1984;141(1): 136-7.*

[102] *Mitsuyama,Y.,Kogoh, H. Serum and cerebrospinal fluid vitamin B12 levels in demented patients with CH3-B12 treatment-preliminary study. Japanese Journal of Psychiatry and Neurology ,1988; 42(1):65-71.*

[103] *Van Tiggelen, C.J.M., Peperkamp, J.P.C., TerToolen, J.F.W. Vitamin - B12 levels of cerebrospinal fluid in patients with organic mental disorder. Journal of Orthomolecular Psychiatry, 1983, 12:305-11.*

[104] *Donaldson MS Metabloic Vitamin B12 Status on a Mostly Raw Vegan Diet with Follow-Up Using Tablets, Nutrtional Yeast, or Probiotic Supplements. Ann Nutr Metab 2000;44:229-234.*

[105] *Crane MG, Register UD, Lukens RH, Gregory R. Cobalamin (CBL) studies on two total vegetarian (vegan) families. Vegetarian Nutr Int J 1998; 2/3: 87-92.*

[106] *Matchar DB, Feussner JR, Millington DS, et al. Isotope dilution assay for urinary methylmalonic acid in the diagnosis of vitamin B12 deficiency-*

A prospective clinical evaluation. Ann Intern Med 1987; 106: 707-710.

[107] *Yamauchi H, Omine M, Tsukamoto N, et al. Urinary methylmalonic acid excretion and clinical features in megaloblastic anemia due to vitamin B12 deficiency. Jpn J Clin Hematol 1989; 30:835-839.*

[108] *Anand A. Urinary methylmalonic acid and cobalamin deficiency in the elderly. Am J Med 1995; 98:514.*

[109] *Norman EJ, Cronin C. Cobalamin deficiency. Neurology 1996; 47: 310-311.*

[110] *Test ID: MMAS:Methylmalonic Acid (MMA), Quantitative, Serum, Mayo Medical Laboritories, Avaialable at: http:// www.mayomedicallaboratories.com/test-catalog/Clinical+and +Interpretive/80289, Retrieved on: 2012.06.03.*

[111] *Test ID: MMAU80290:Methylmalonic Acid (MMA), Quantitative, Urine, Mayo Medical Laboratories, Available at :http:// www.mayomedicallaboratories.com/test-catalog/print/80290. Retrieved on: 2012.06.03*

[112] *Loehrer FM, Schwab R, Angst CP, Haefeli WE, Fowler B. Influence of oral S-adenosylmethionine on plasma 5-methyltetrahydrofolate, S-adenosylhomocysteine, homocysteine and methionine in healthy humans. J Pharmacol Exp Ther. 1997 Aug;282(2):845-50.*

[113] *McBride, J., 2000, B12 Deficiency May Be More Widespread Than Thought, Available at : http://www.ars.usda.gov/is/pr/2000/000802.htm (May 4,2012).*

[114] *http://www.b12d.org/content/what-vitamin-b12*

[115] *http://www.b12d.org/content/different-types-b12*

[116] *http://www.b12d.org/content/vitamin-b12-%E2%80%93-your-daily-dose*

[117] *Institute of Medicine. Food and Nutrition Board. Dietary Reference Intakes: Thiamin, Riboflavin, Niacin, Vitamin B6, Folate, Vitamin B12, Pantothenic Acid, Biotin, and Choline. Washington, DC: National Academy Press, 1998.*

[118] *Carmel R. How I treat cobalamin (vitamin B12) deficiency. Blood. 2008;112:2214-21.*

[119] *ttp://ods.od.nih.gov/factsheets/VitaminB12-HealthProfessional/*

[120] *Yazaki Y, Chow G, Mattie M. A single-center, double-blinded, randomized controlled study to evaluate the relative efficacy of sublingual and oral vitamin B-complex administration in reducing total serum homocysteine levels. J Altern Complement Med 2006;12:881-5.*

[121] *Sharabi A, Cohen E, Sulkes J, Garty M. Replacement therapy for vitamin B12 deficiency: comparison between the sublingual and oral route. Br J Clin Pharmacol 2003;56:635-8.*

[122] *http://www.b12d.org/content/buying-vitamin-b12-supplements*

[123] *Andrès E, Federici L, Affenberger S, Vidal-Alaball J, Loukili NH, Zimmer J, et al. B12 deficiency: a look beyond pernicious anemia. J Fam Pract 2007;56:537-42.*

[124] *Suzuki DM, Alagiakrishnan K, Masaki KH, Okada A, Carethers M. Patient acceptance of intranasal cobalamin gel for vitamin B12 replacement therapy. Hawaii Med J 2006;65:311-4.*

[125] *Slot WB, Merkus FW, Van Deventer SJ, Tytgat GN. Normalization of plasma vitamin B12 concentration by intranasal hydroxocobalamin in vitamin B12-deficient patients. Gastroenterology.1997;113:430-3.*

[126] *http://en.allexperts.com/q/Lupus-2910/2009/4/lupus-2.htm*

[127] *http://www.b12patch.com/blog/autoimmune-disease/if-vitamin-b12-deficiency-mimics-multiple-sclerosis-how-do-you-tell-the-difference/*

[128] *http://chriskresser.com/b12-deficiency-a-silent-epidemic-with-serious-consequences*

[129] *http://www.b12d.org/content/cost-mis-diagnosis*